Gratitude

30 day

guided journal

by trina kay

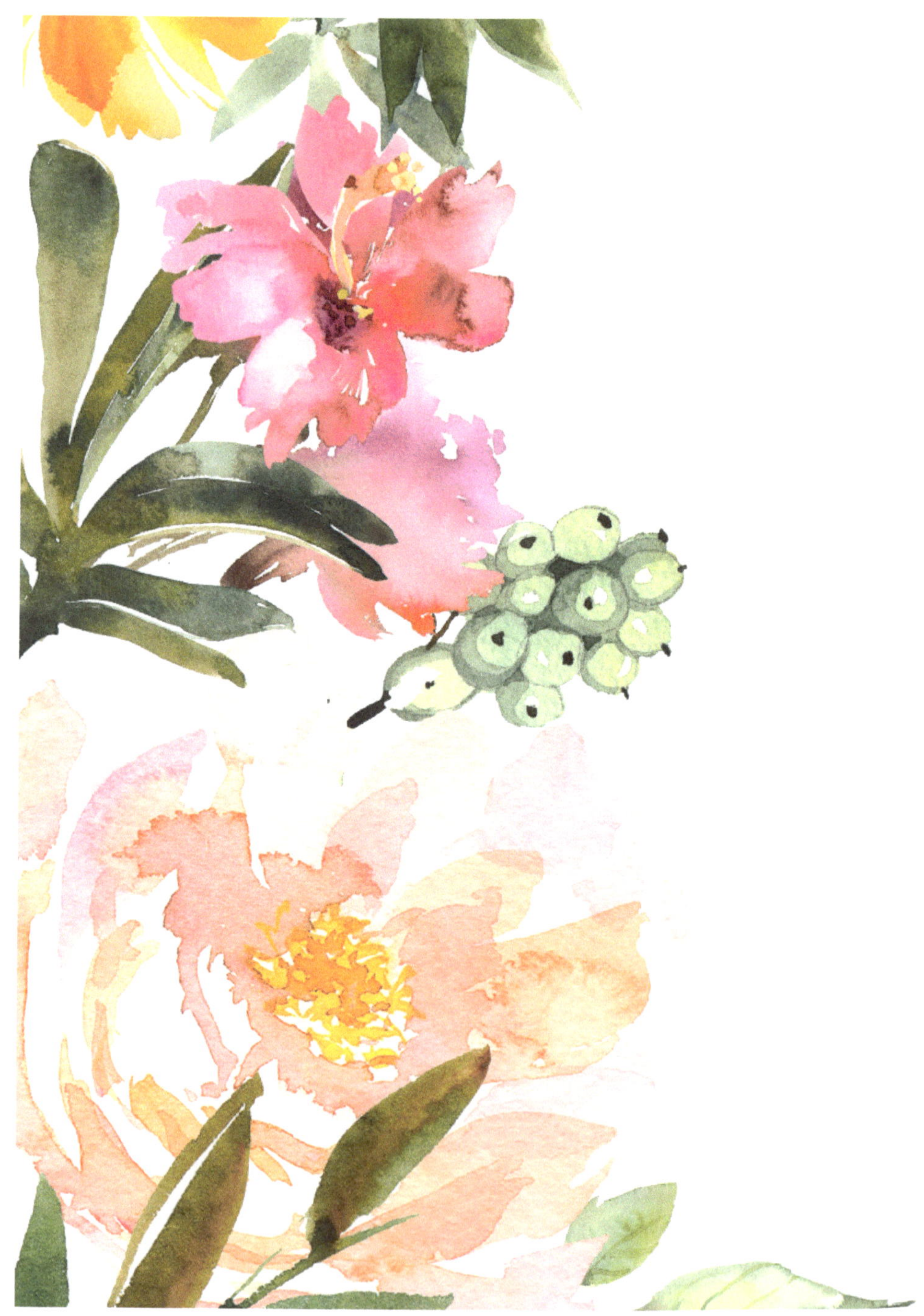

This
book
belongs
to :

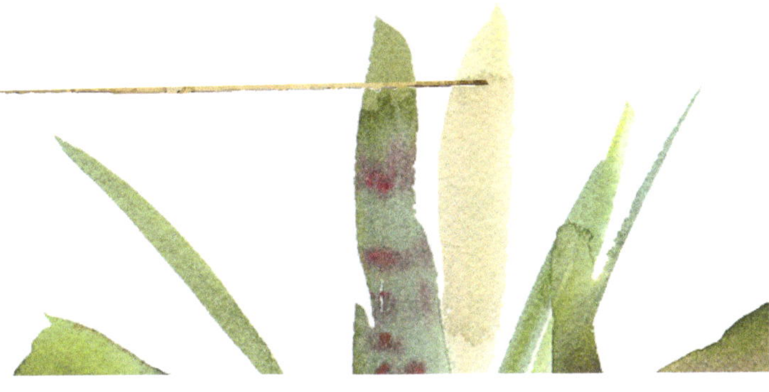

Thank you, Cherry, for teaching me how to mindfully appreciate each moment.

ISBN: 9798732654783

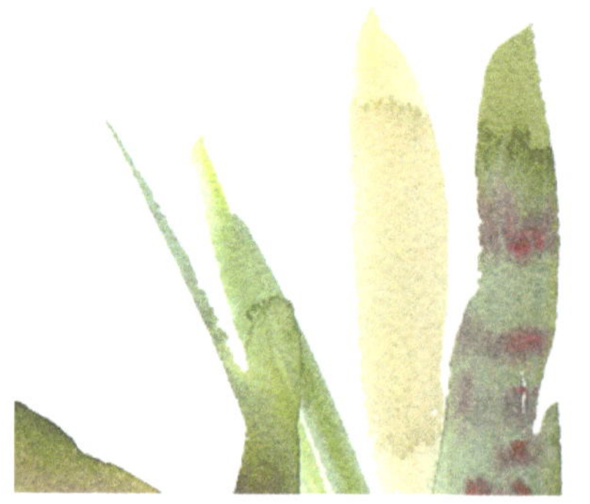

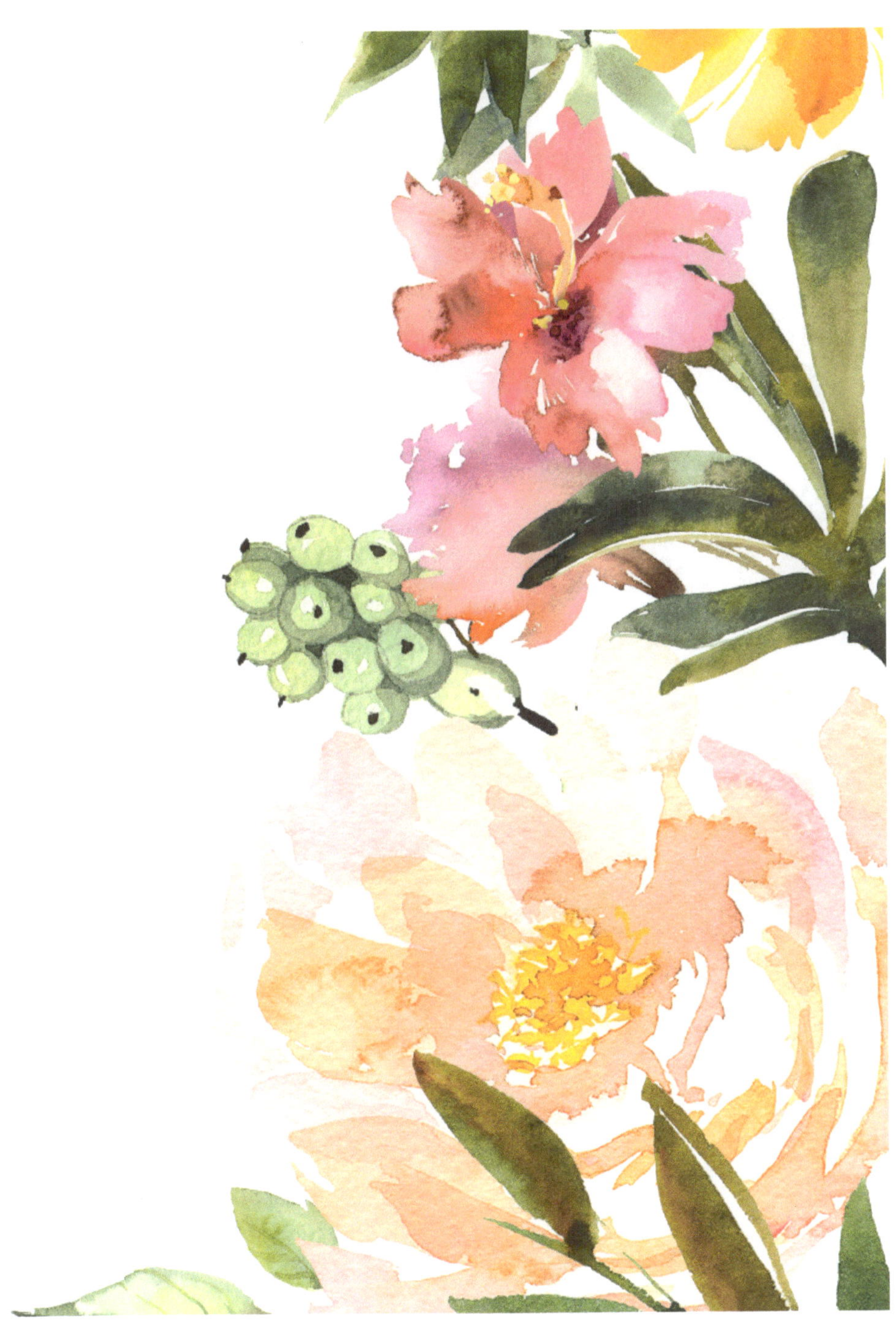

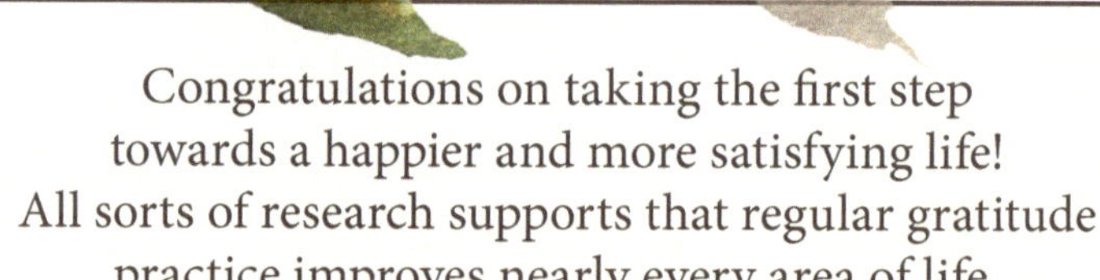

Congratulations on taking the first step
towards a happier and more satisfying life!
All sorts of research supports that regular gratitude
practice improves nearly every area of life.

It's not going to be easy, but you can do it.

Whenever you're ready, spend just five minutes each
day to noticing things in your life you appreciate
then write them down in this journal.
Just before bed is best for me.
You do what works best for you.

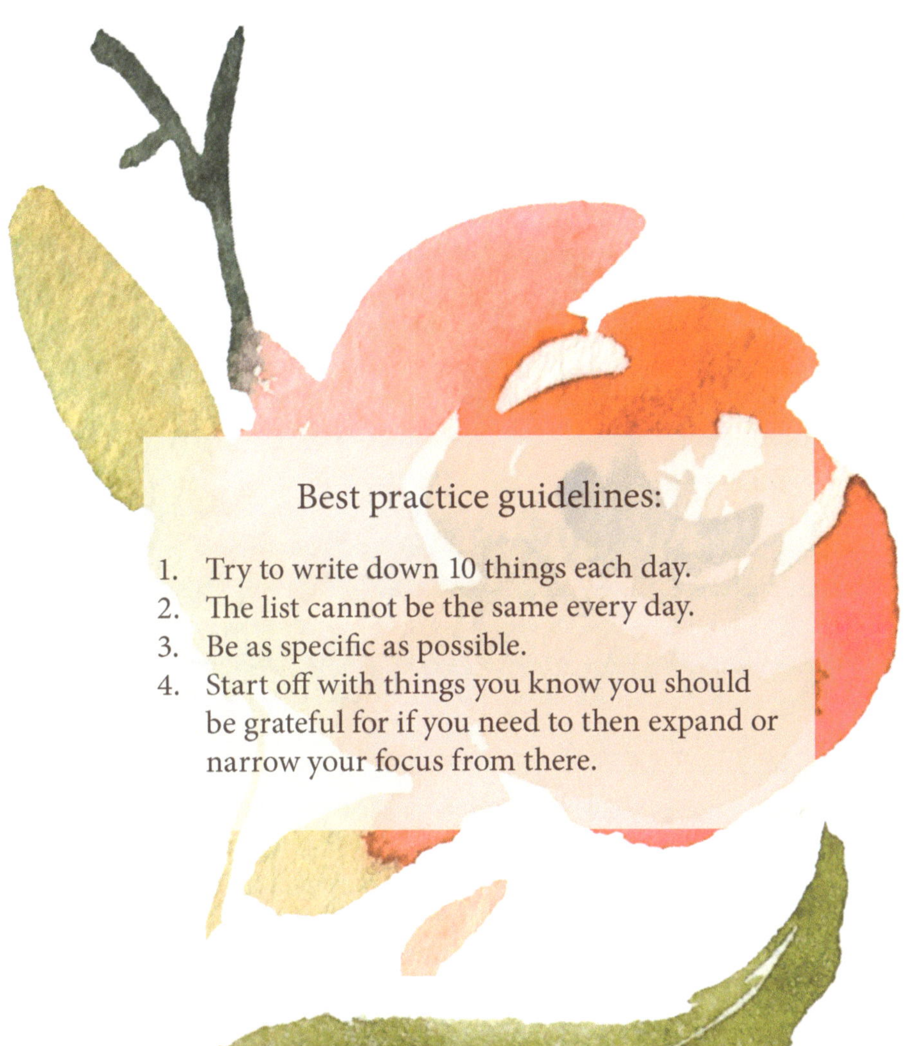

Best practice guidelines:

1. Try to write down 10 things each day.
2. The list cannot be the same every day.
3. Be as specific as possible.
4. Start off with things you know you should be grateful for if you need to then expand or narrow your focus from there.

Day 1

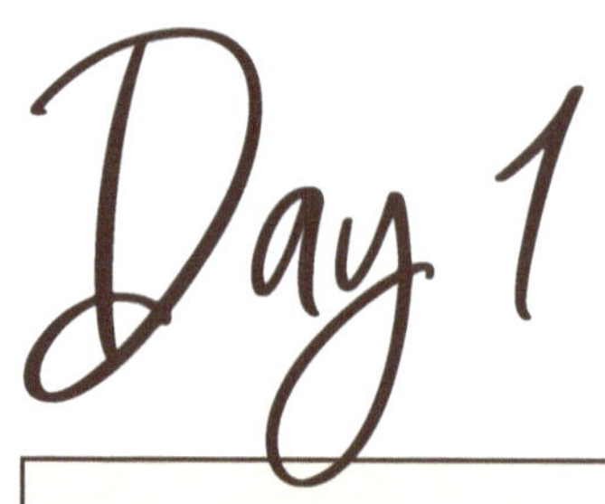

What person from your past had a positive influence in shaping you into the person you are today?

What do you appreciate most about them? What has thier teaching helped you accomplish?

Regular gratitude practice combats the negative thinking patterns we developed over time by focusing on wants that never satisfied or by comparing ourselves to others. Both from the perspective of scarcity or personal lacking.

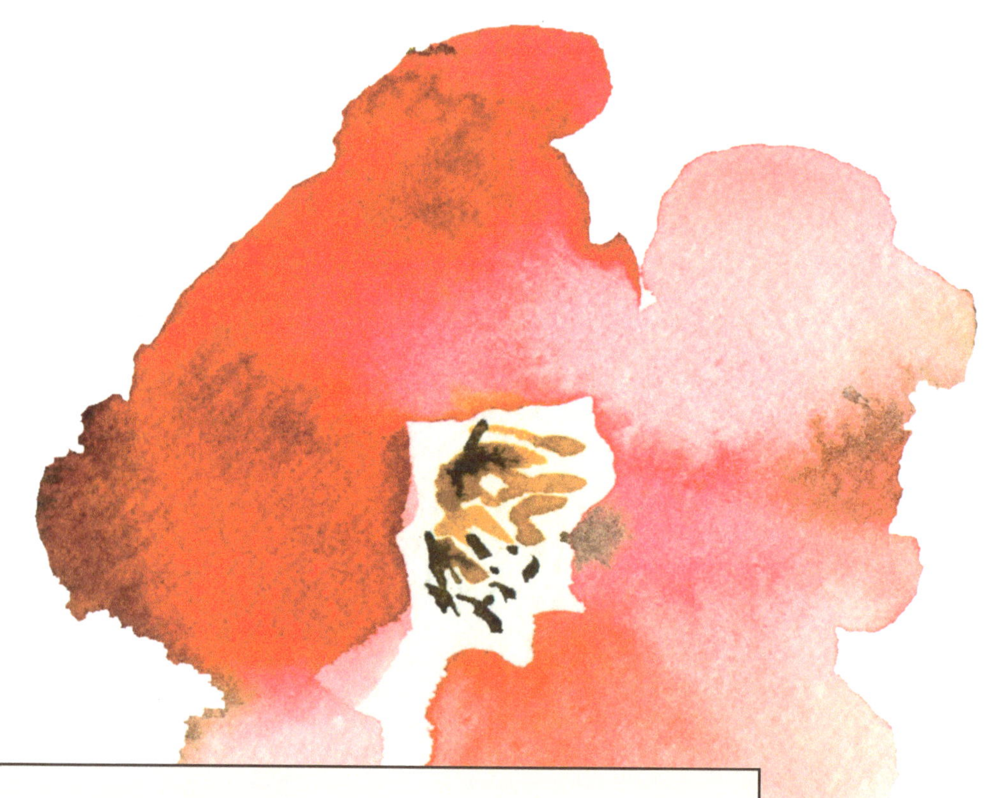

A simple shift from a perspective of
scarcity to one of appreciation opens
your mind to see wonder and abundance
everywhere you look. Just wait and see.
You are already gaining momentum.

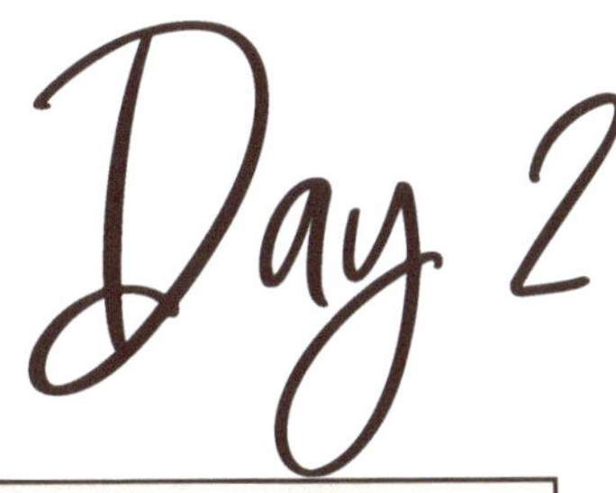

What unexpected pleasure did you experience today?

Perhaps the smell of rain? A rainbow? A stranger whose smile was contagious? Knowing your smile was contagious?

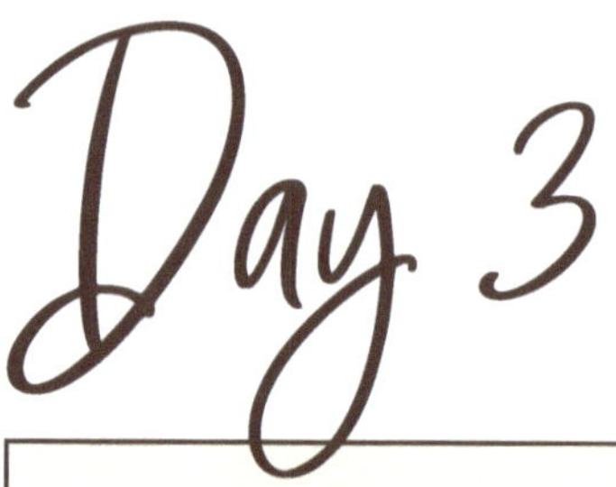

Day 3

What delighted your senses today?

A painting that sparks joy for you? The smell of magnolias wafting in the breeze? Luxurious hand lotion? Jazz?

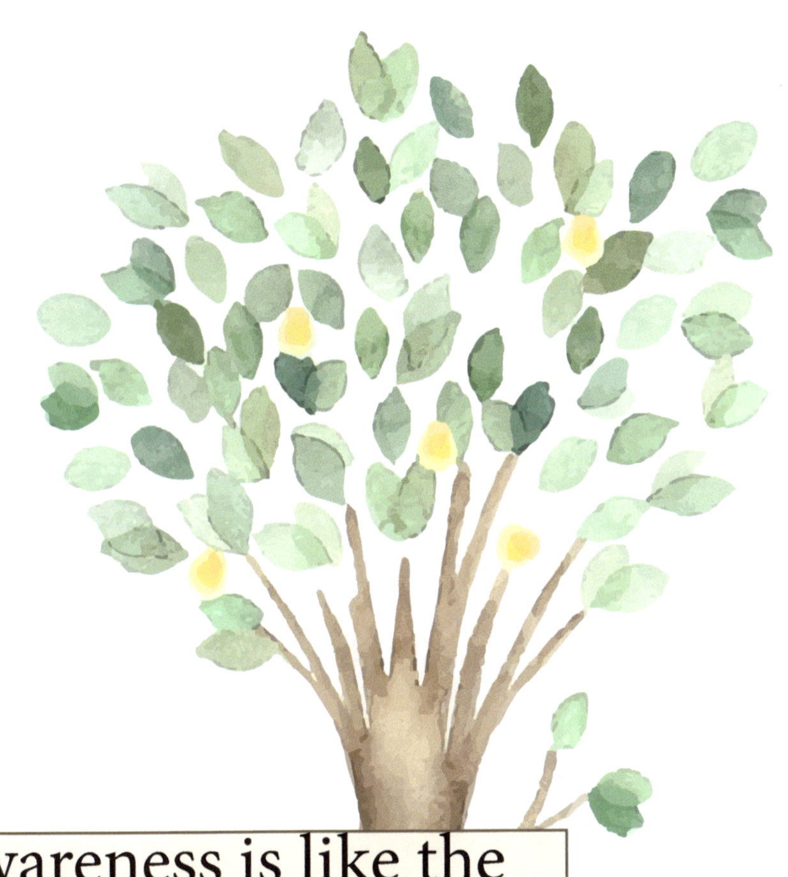

"Awareness is like the sun. When it shines on things, they are transformed."

- Thich Nhat Hanh

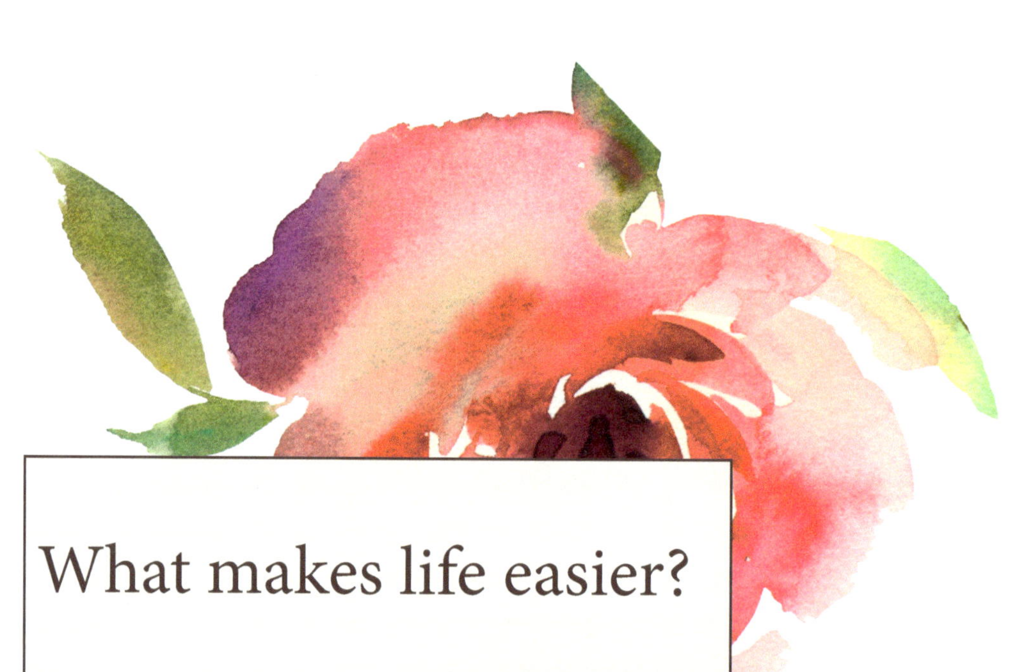
What makes life easier?

Day 4

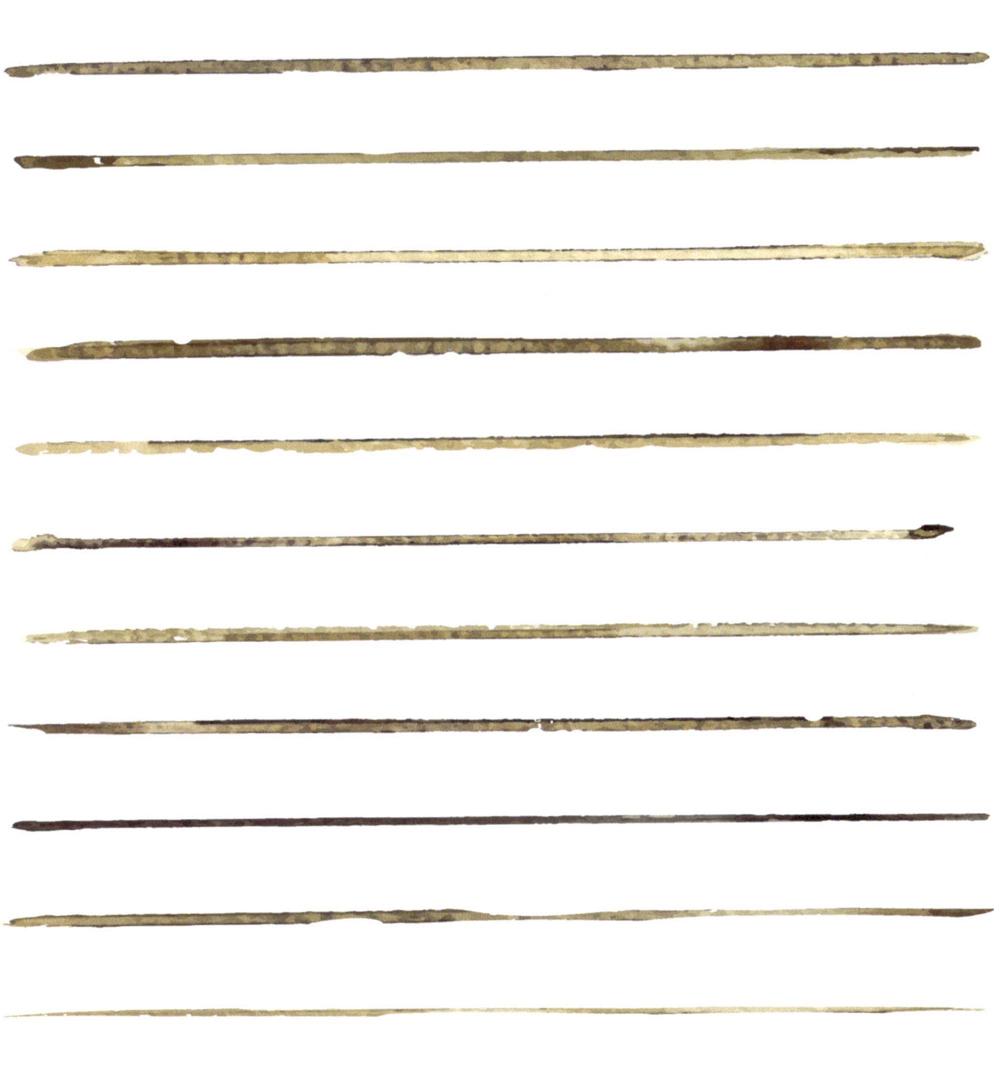

Day 5

What makes life fun?

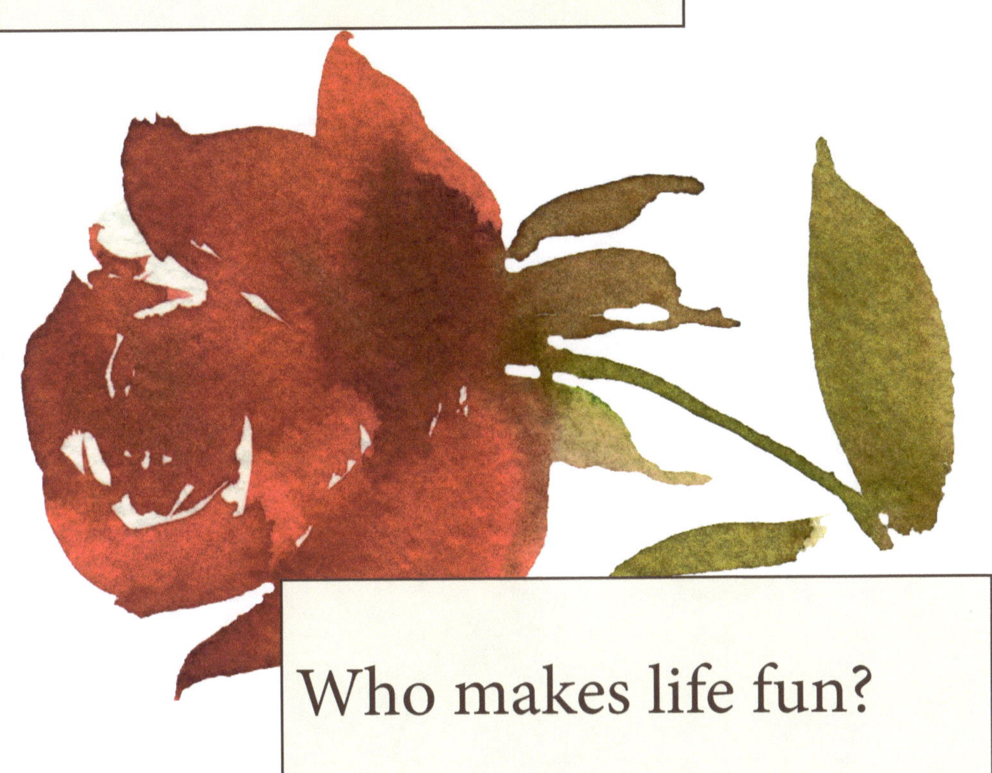

Who makes life fun?

Why or how?

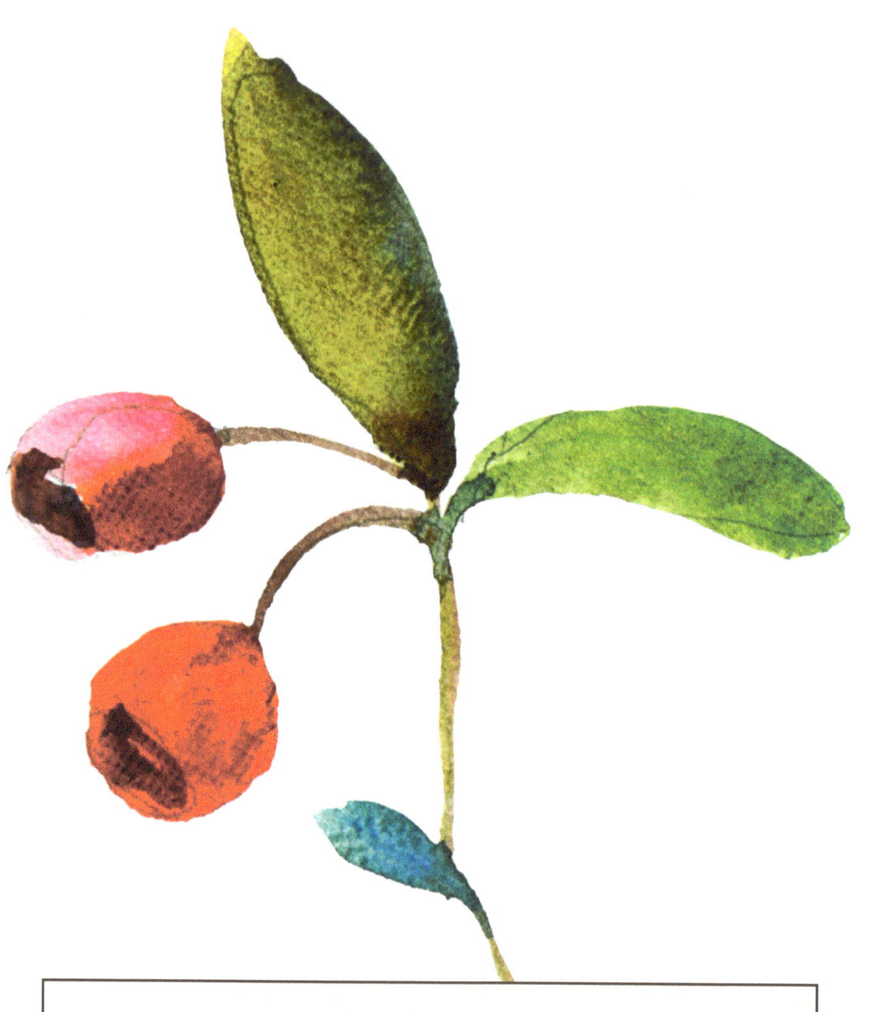

Tell me about the last time
you were on a swing?

Day 6

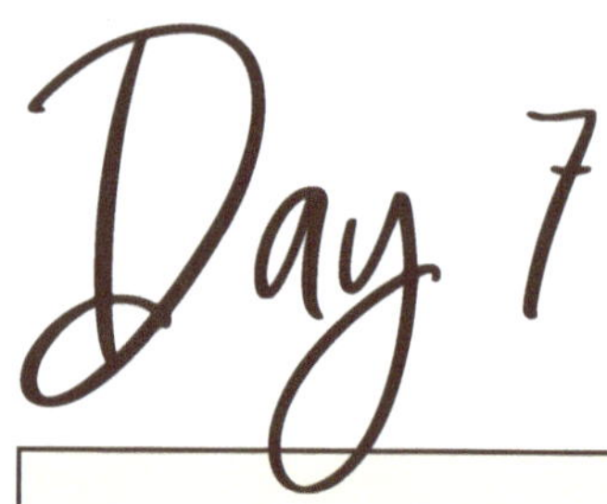

Day 7

Who was the last person that made you laugh?

What made it so funny?

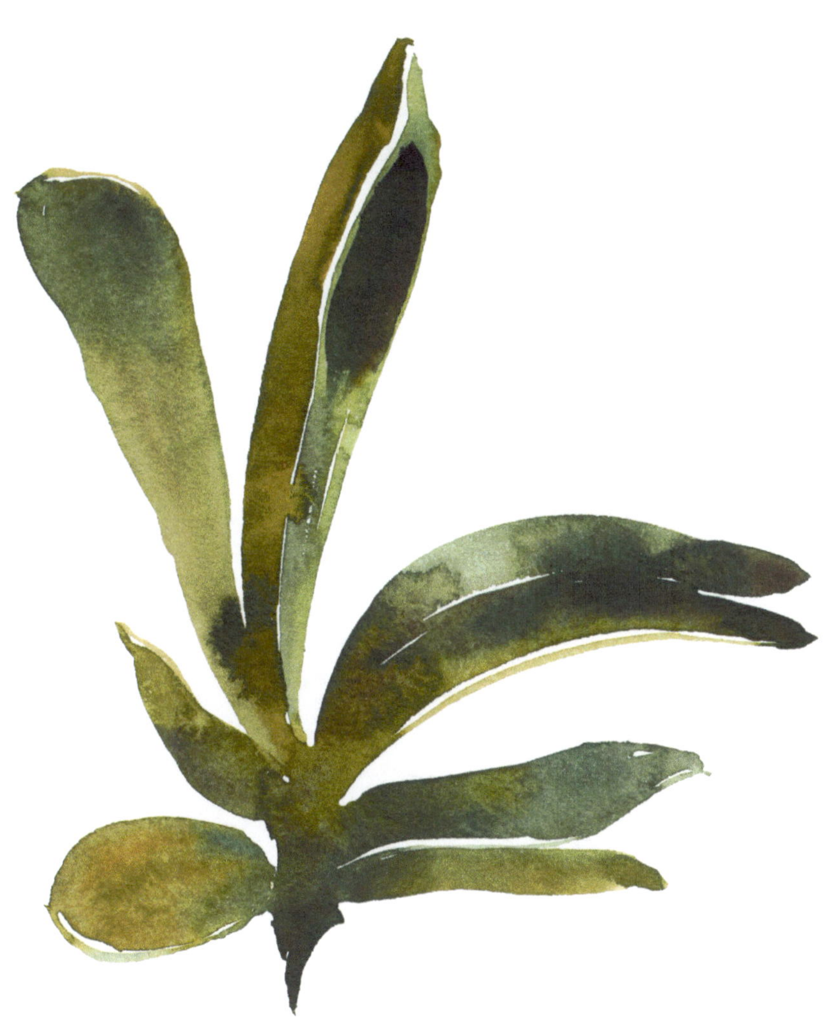

What song makes you smile
every time you hear it?

What makes it special?

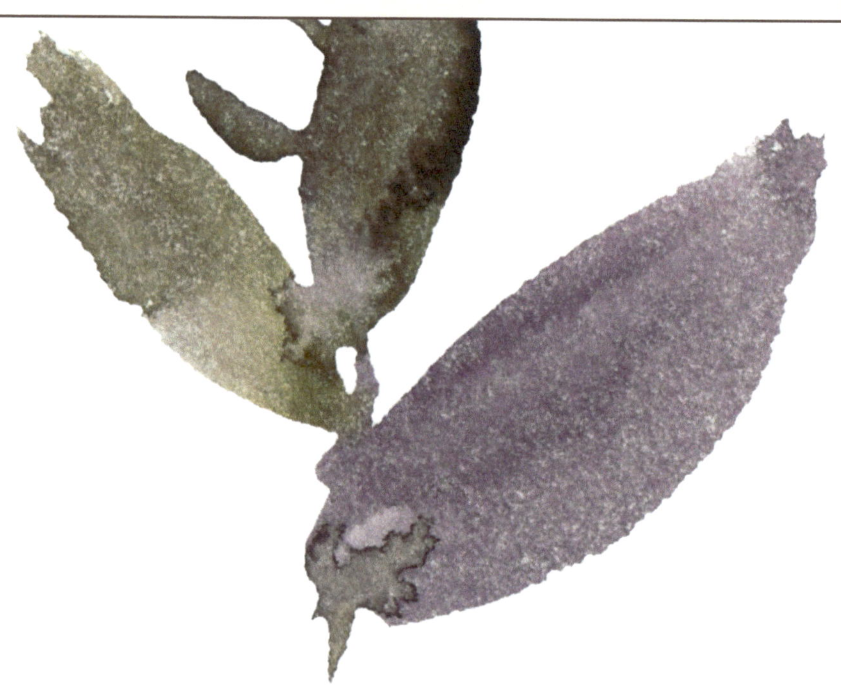

Day 8

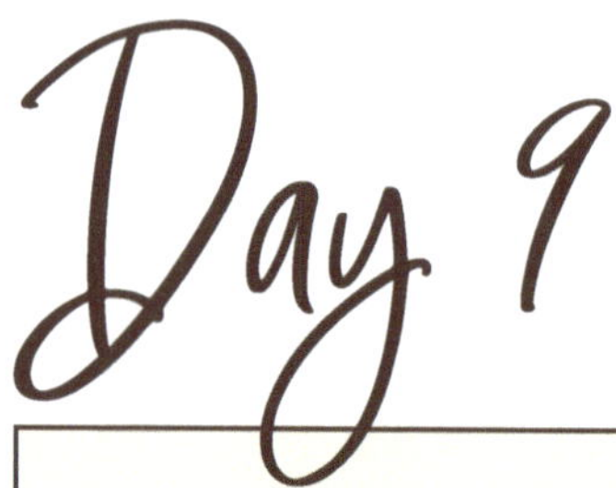

When was the last time you were in awe of nature?

Has a sunset ever brought a tear to your eye?

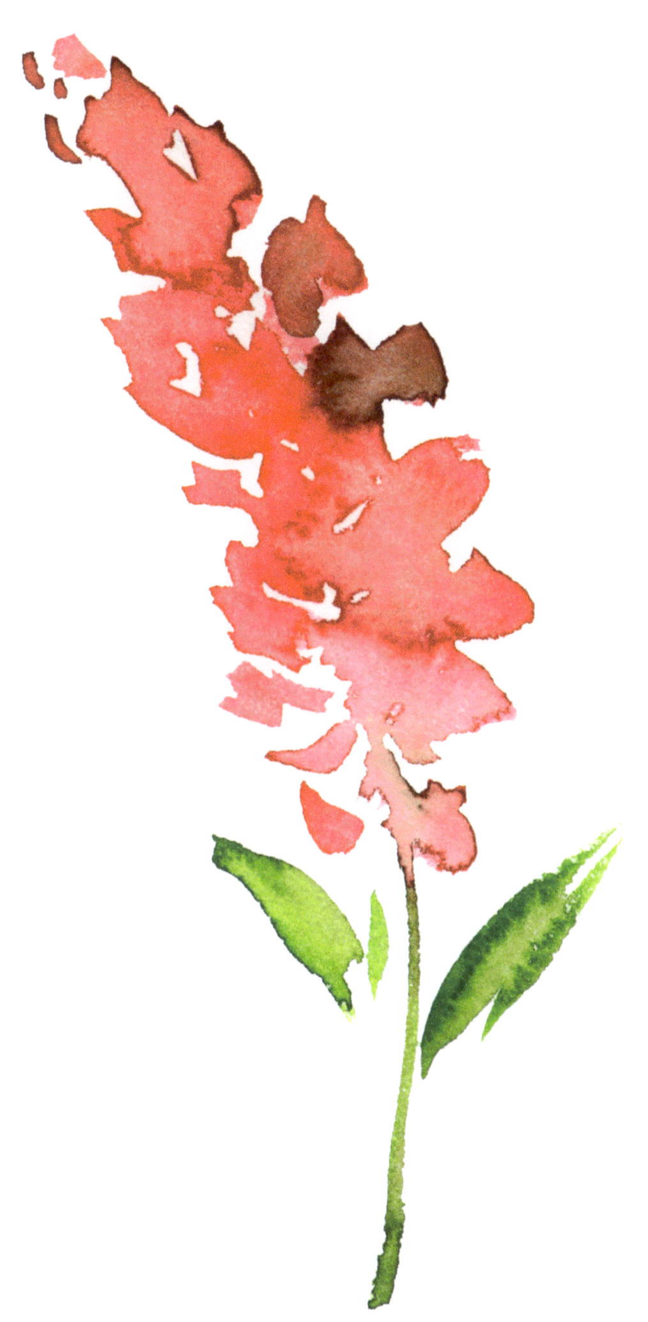

What outfit made you feel beautiful?

Why?

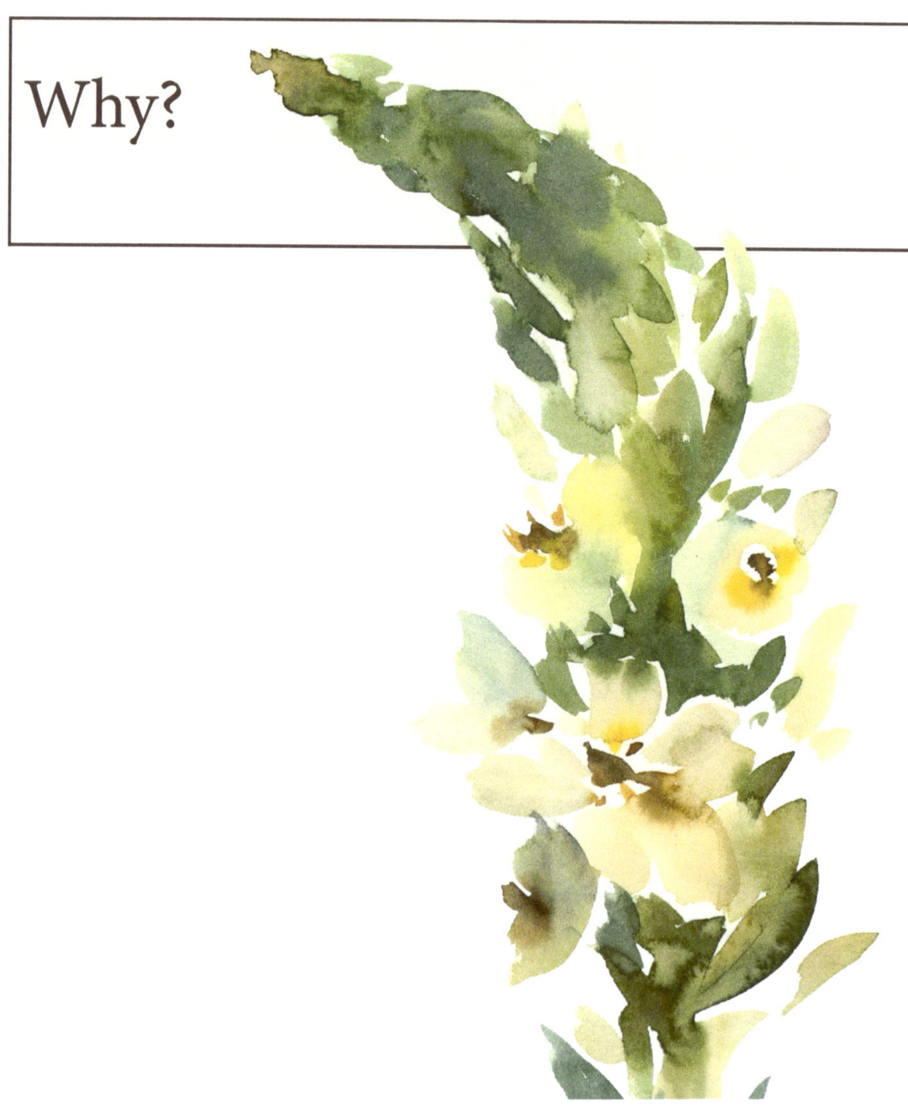

Day 10

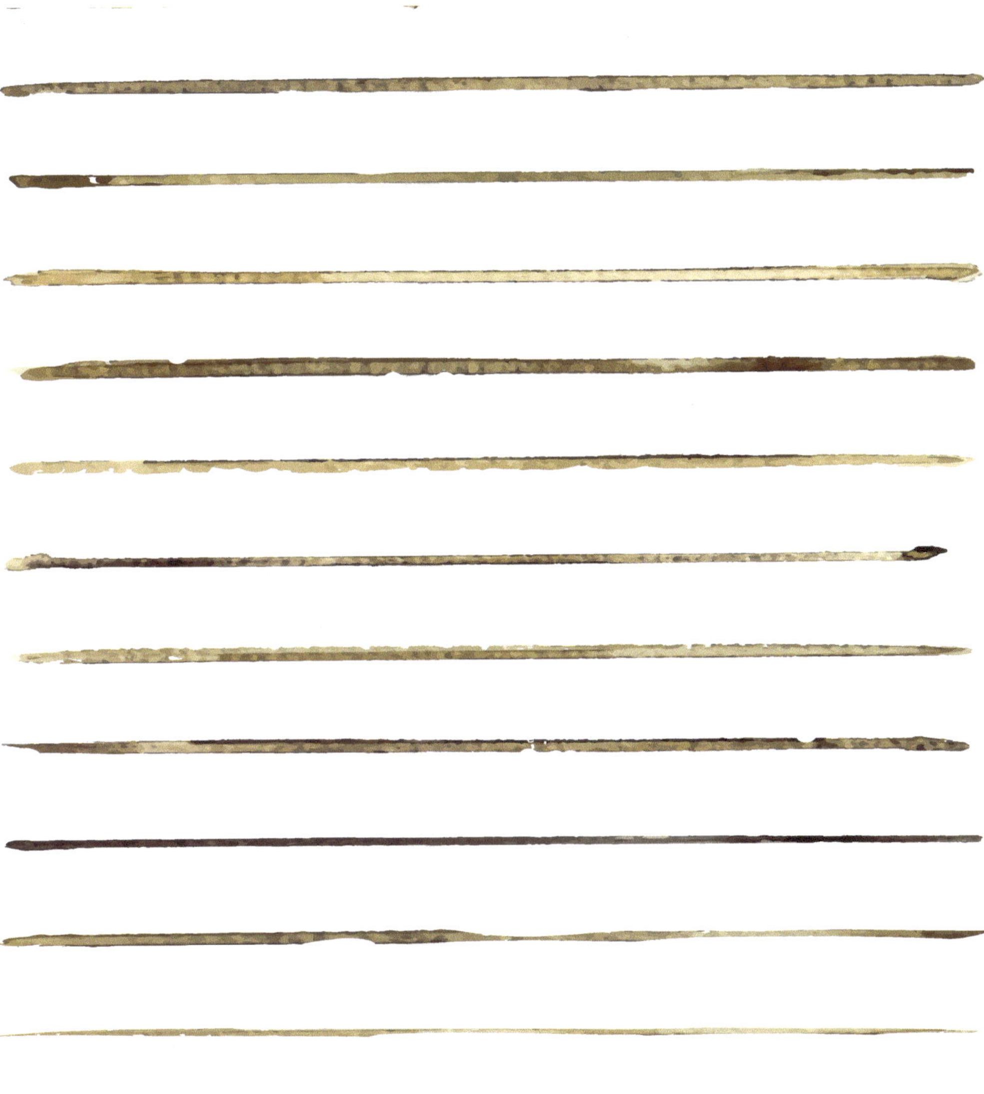

Day 11

What talent or gifting brings you joy when you share it?

How are you blessed by blessing others?

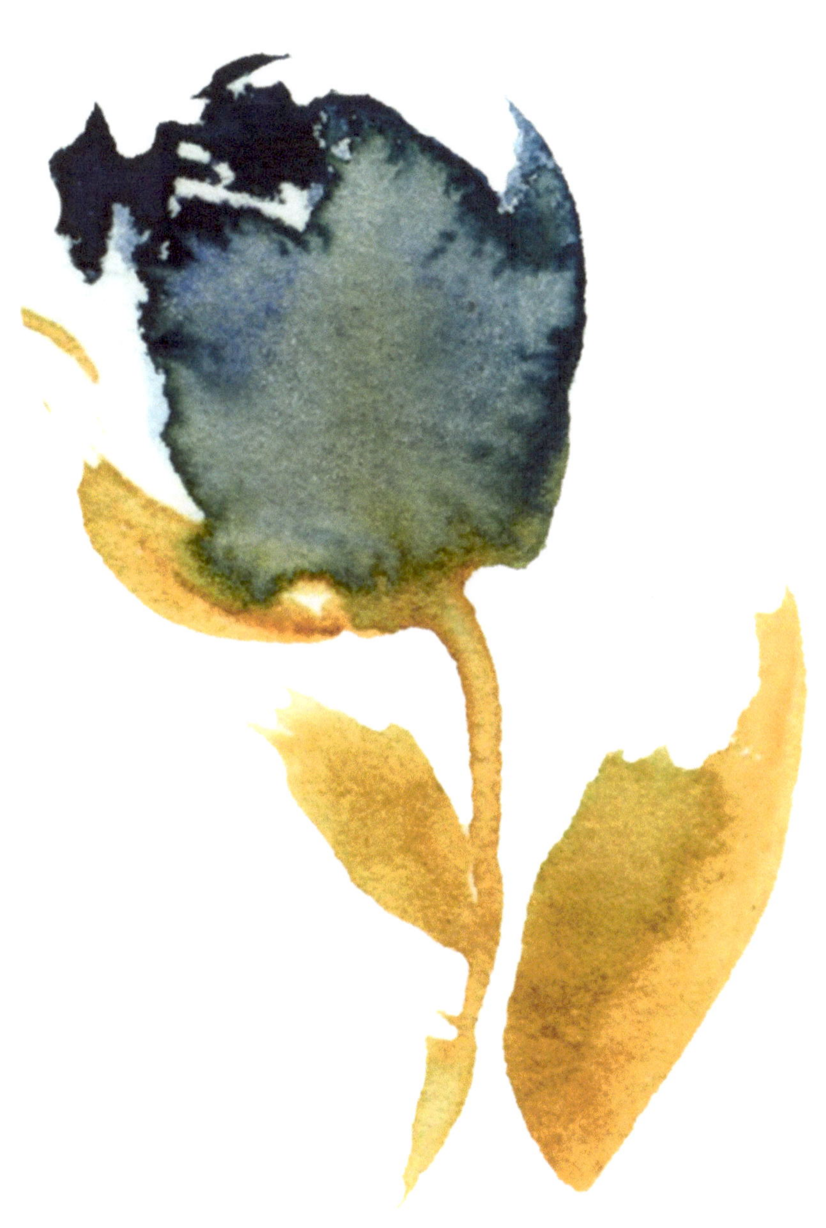

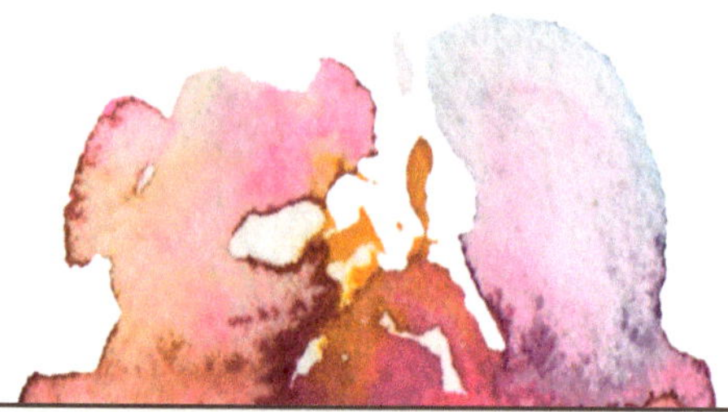

What have you accomplished
you didn't think you could?

How did you do it?

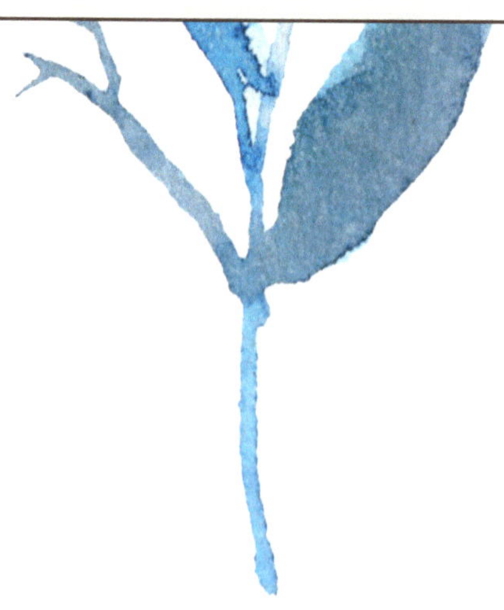

Day 12

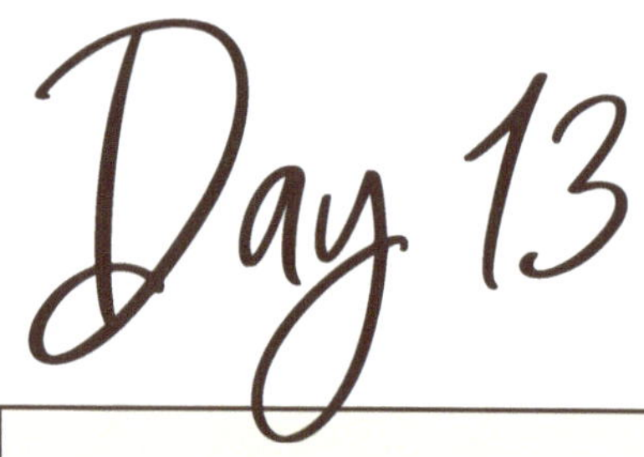

Day 13

What adversity did you overcome?

What can you appreciate about those circumstances?

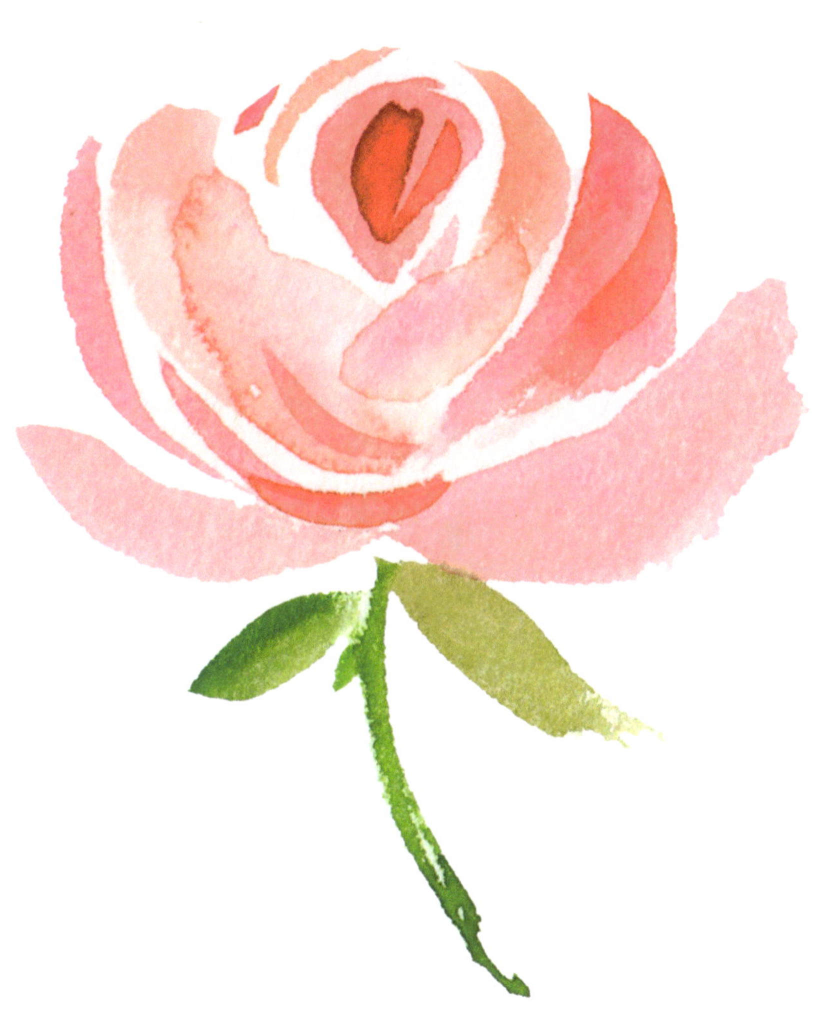

What lessons have you learned from unexpected setbacks?

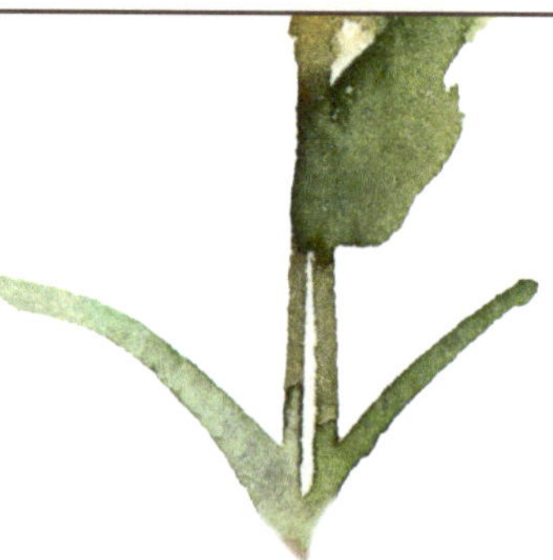

"The last of human freedoms - the ability to chose one's attitude especially an attitude of gratitude in a given set of circumstances especially in difficult circumstances."
Viktor E. Frankl

Day 14

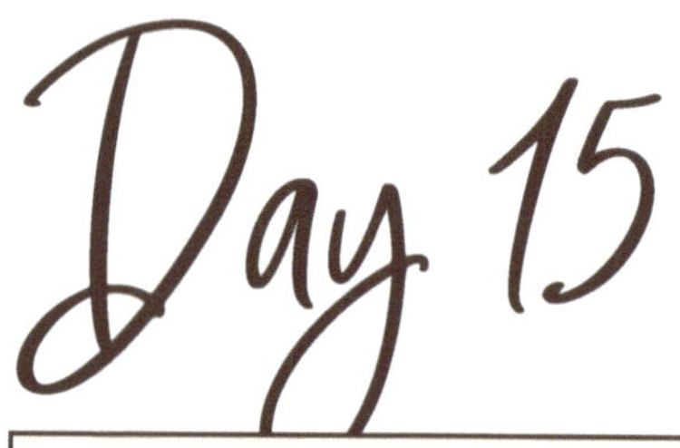

Day 15

What guilty pleasure do you delight in?

Wash away your troubles in a bath full of bubbles.

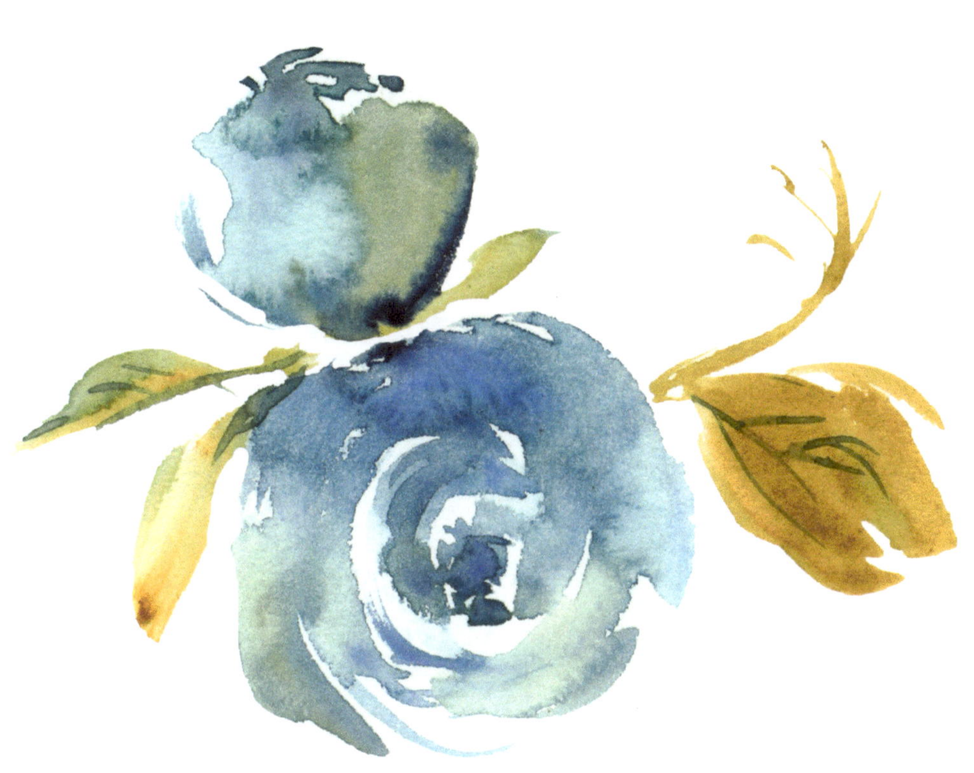

What is your super power?

What makes being you awesome?

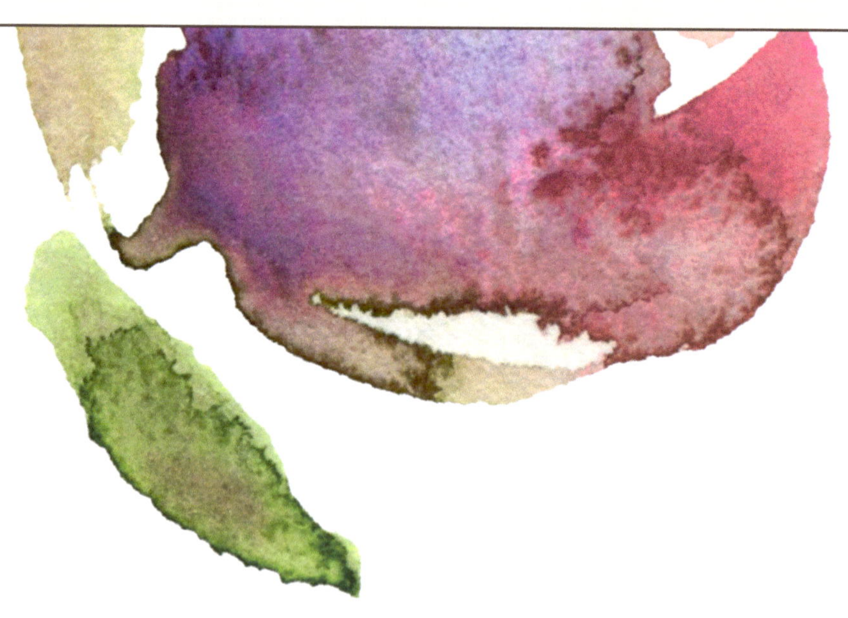

Day 16

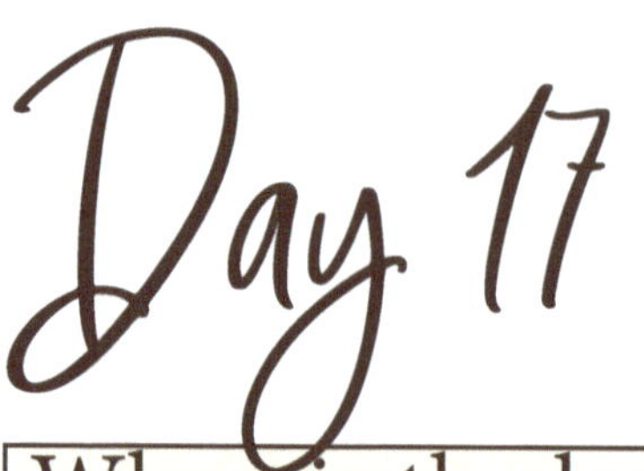

Day 17

When is the last time you stayed up late because your book was too good to put down?

Name a time you were sad because the story ended.

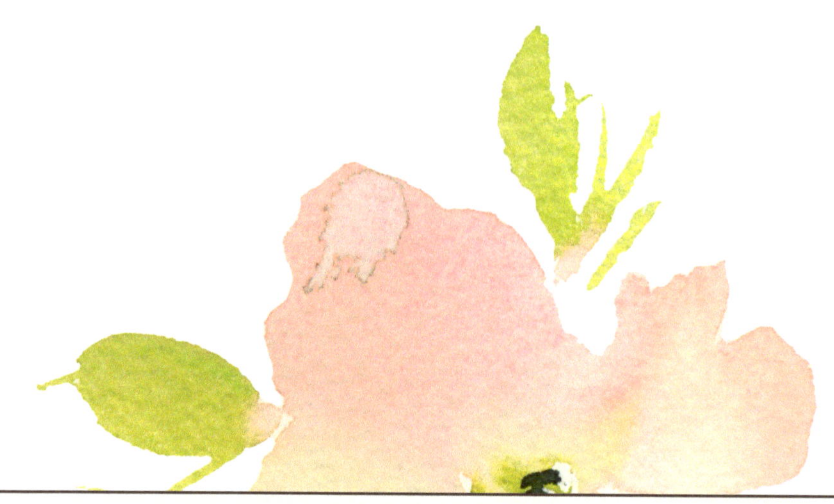

When is the last time you held hands?

Describe how it made you feel.

Day 18

Day 19

When is the last time you were kind to yourself?

How do you nurture your own sweet self?

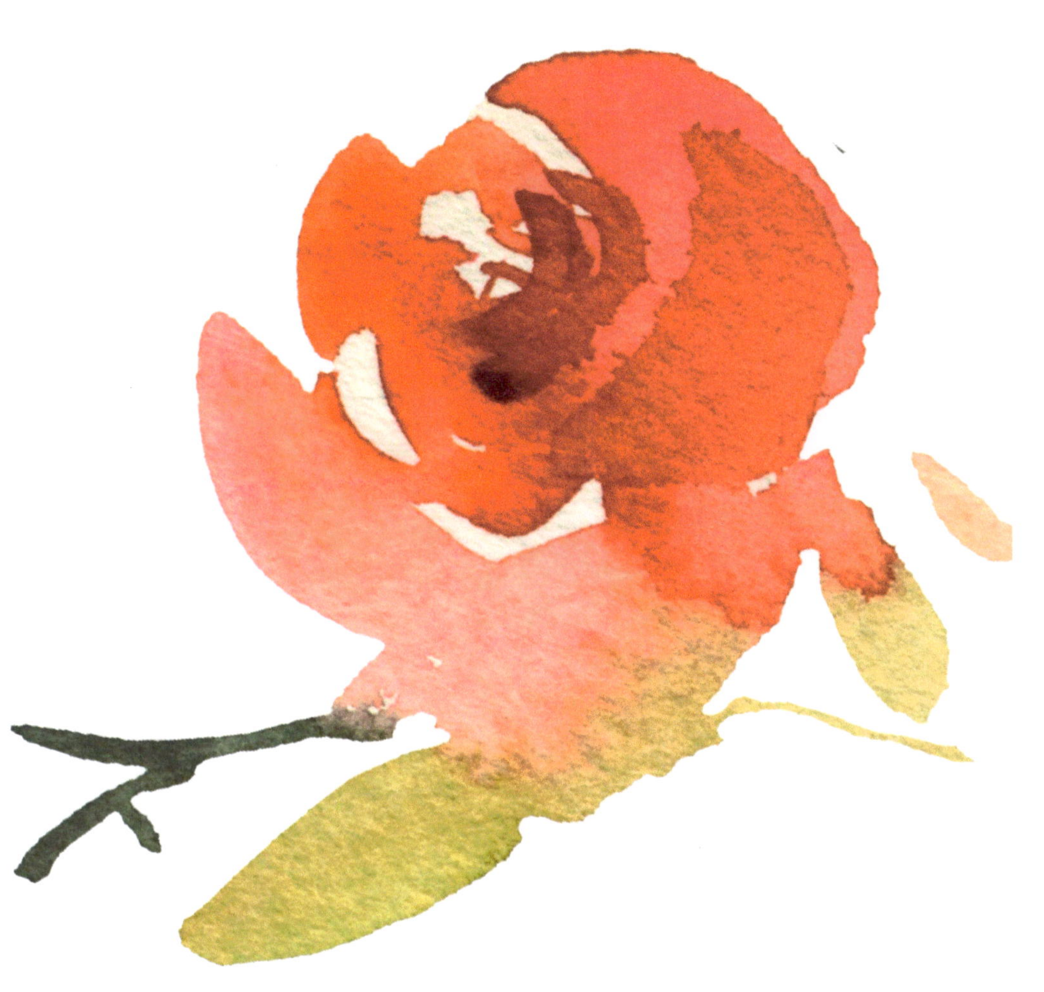

When is the last time you were kind to yourself?

How do you nurture your own sweet self?

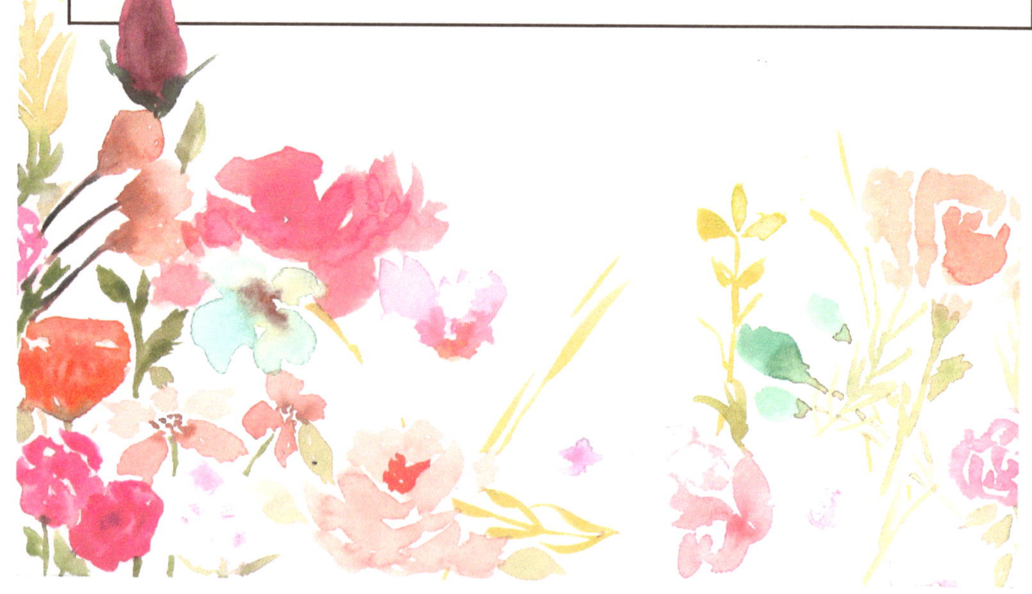

Day 20

Day 21

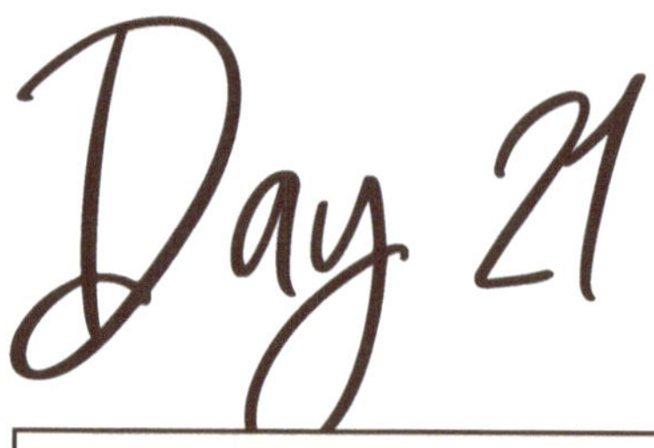

What is the last thing you created?

What do you love about it?

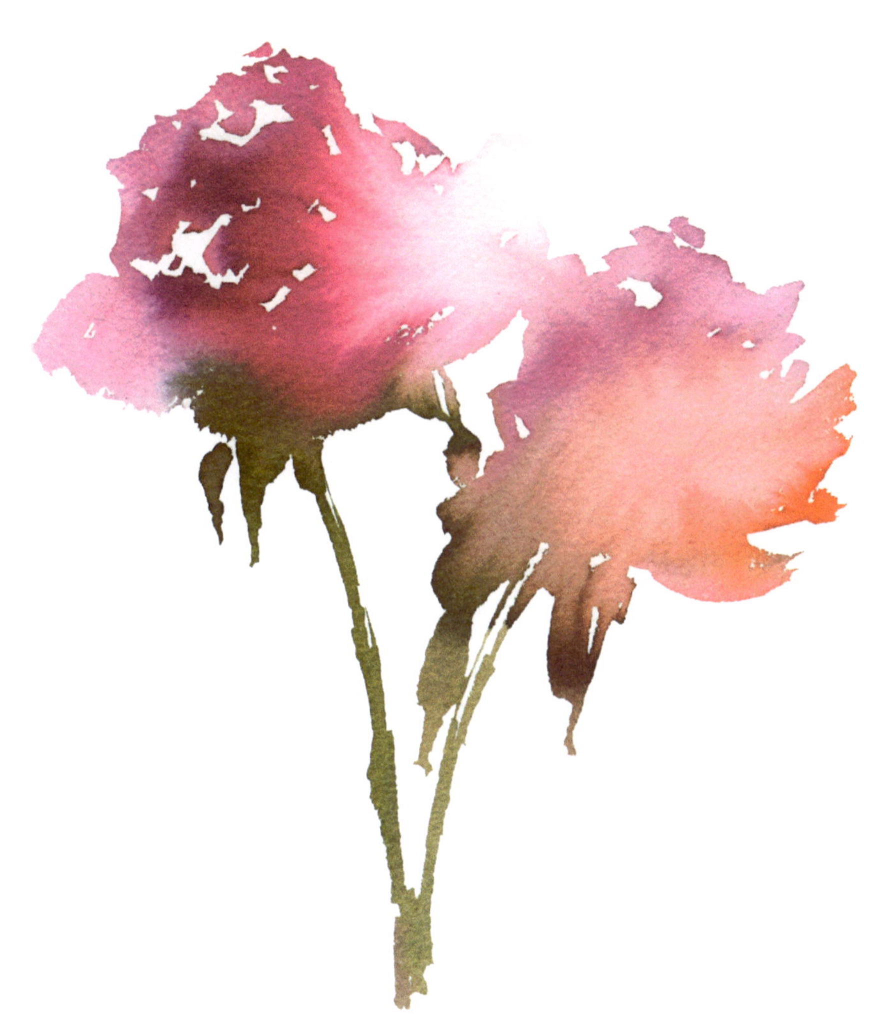

What inspires you?

Who inspires you?

Day 22

Day 23

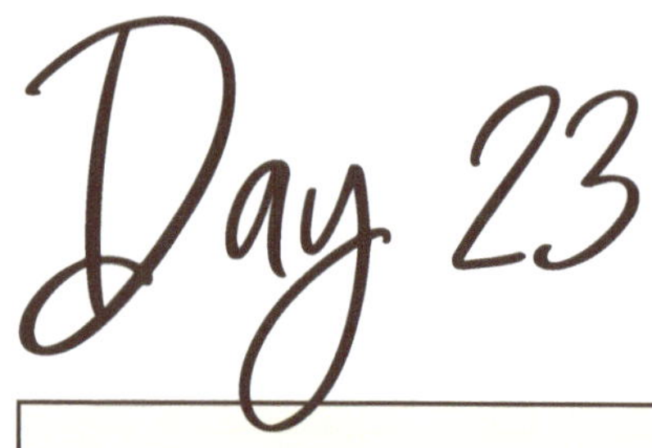

Describe your last spiritual experience?

How did it inform the way you see others?

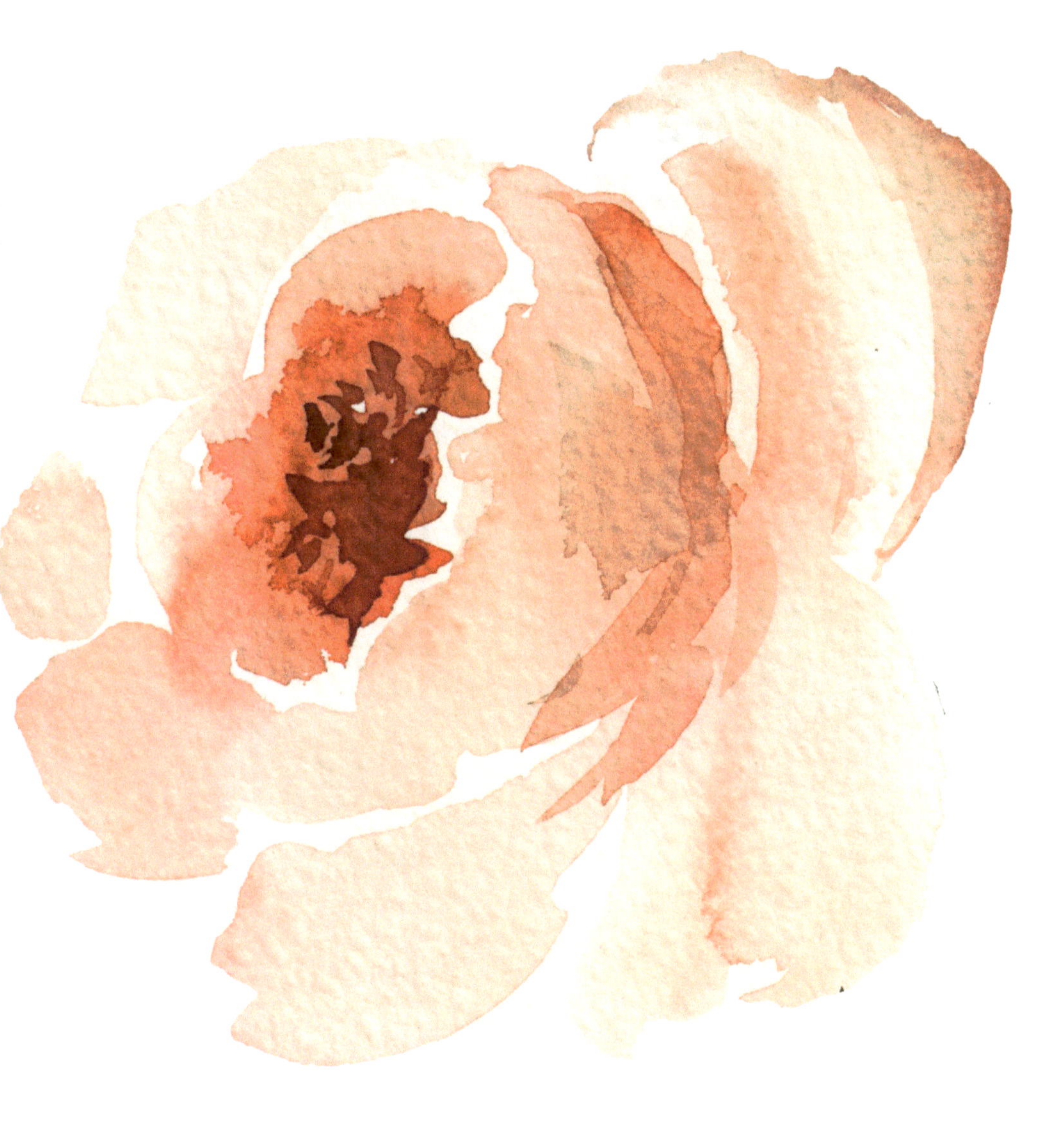

When is the last time you were shown grace you didn't deserve?

How does that impact compassion for others?

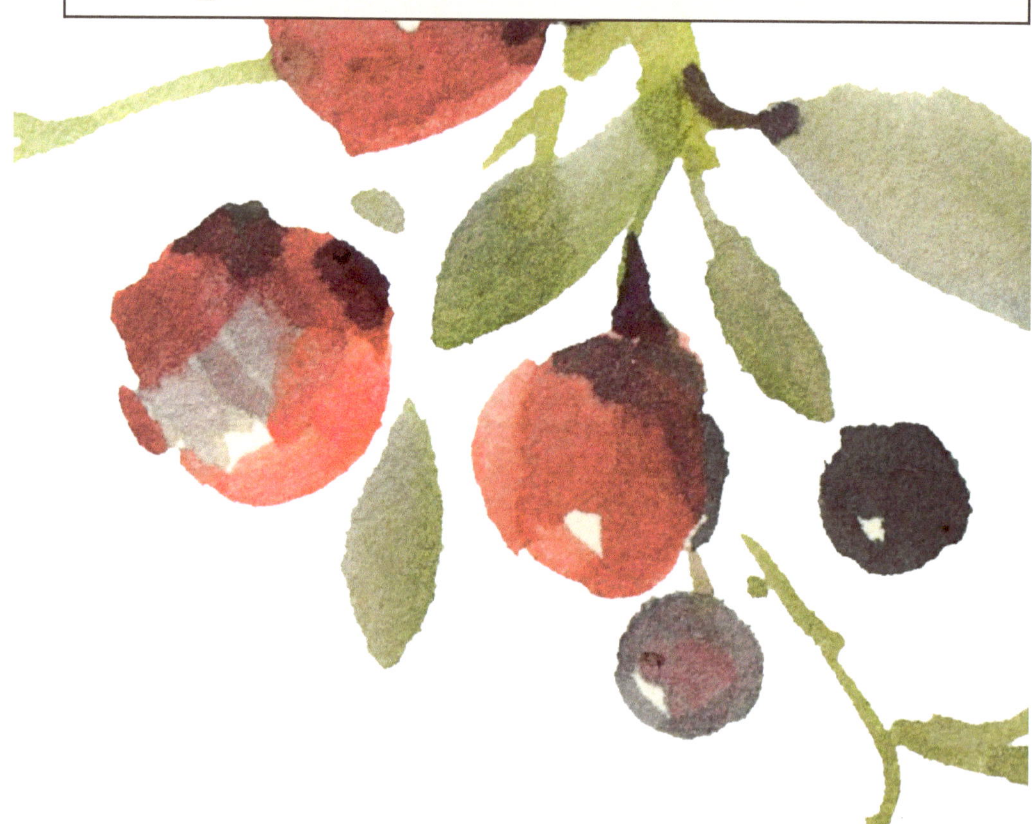

Day 24

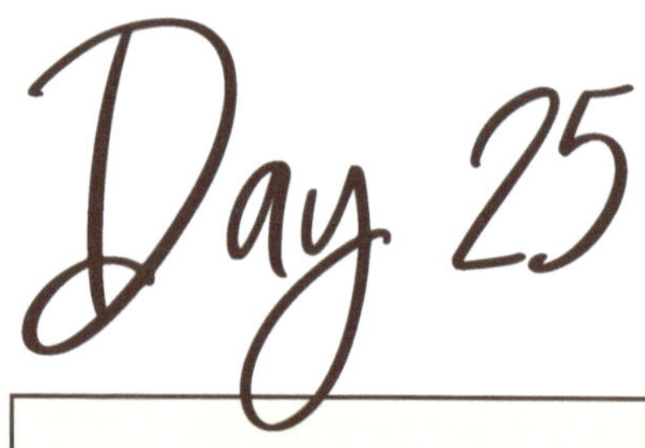

When is the last time you loved with abandon?

What part of the experience did you hide in your heart?

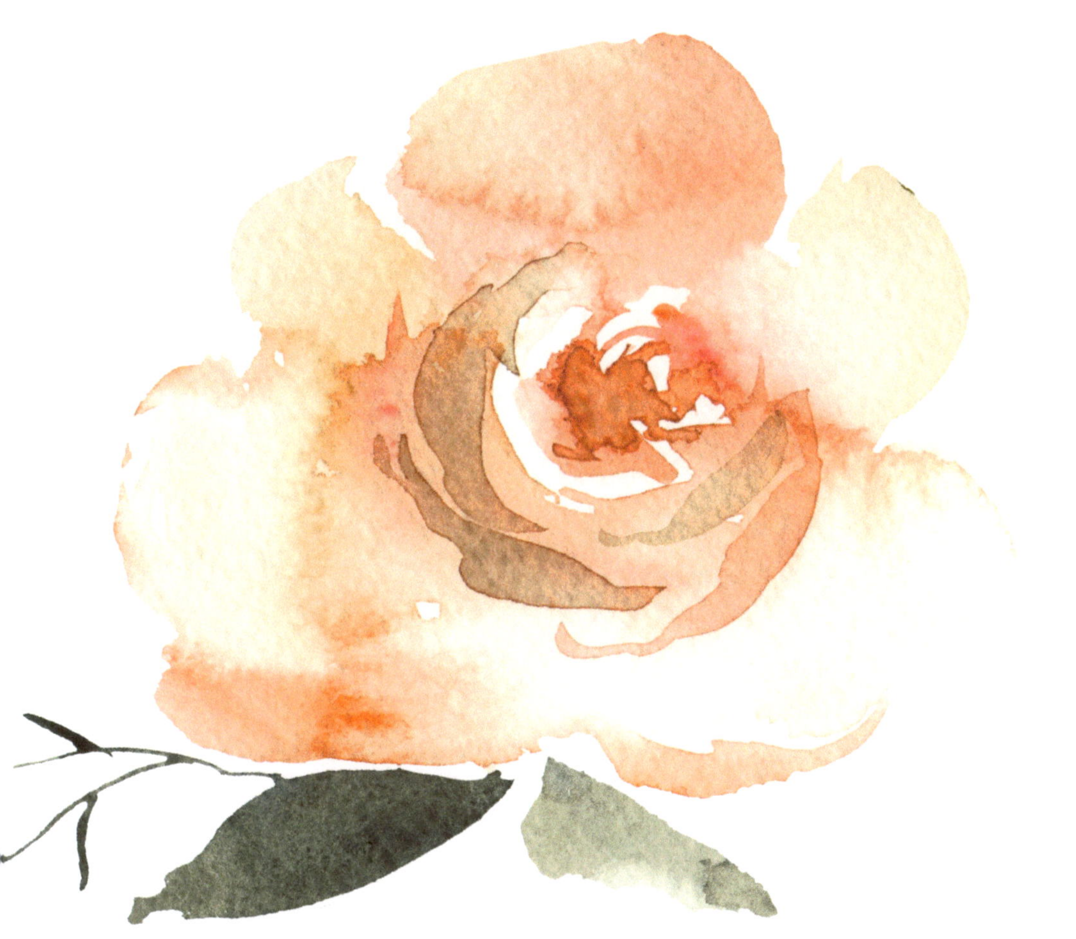

When is the last time you dressed for dinner?

What was the occasion?

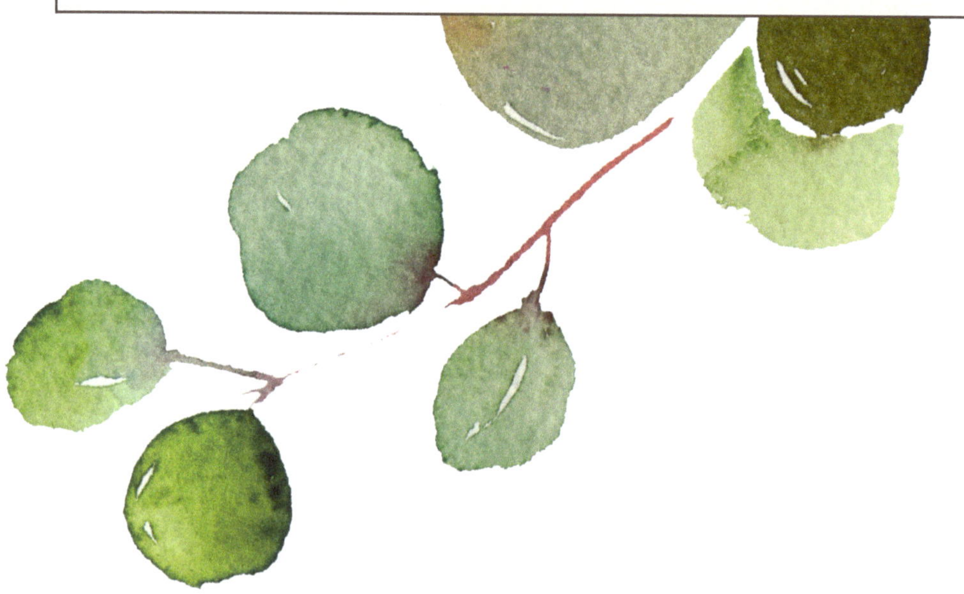

Day 26

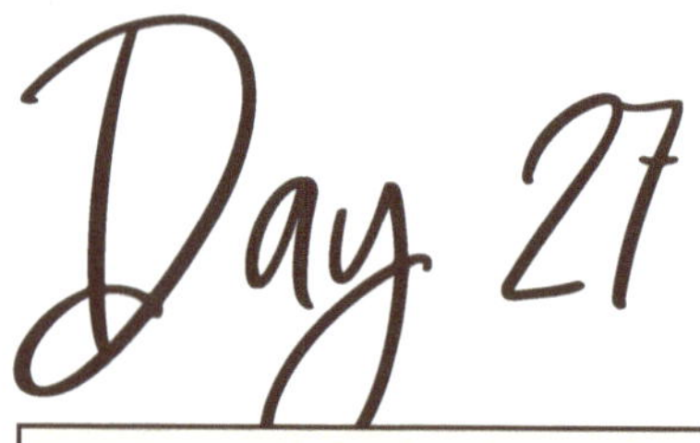

Describe the way sunshine feels on your face.

When is the last time you basked in the sunshine?

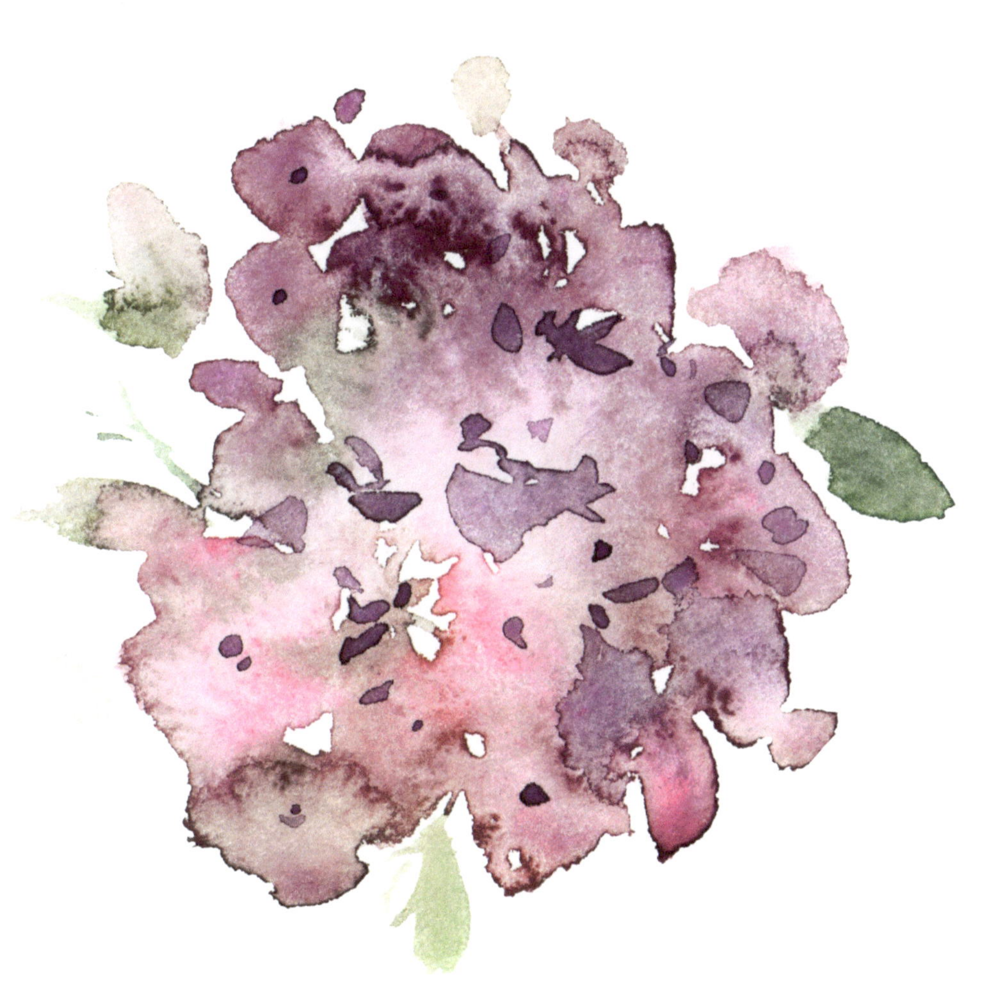

Describe a time when you enjoyed learning about another culture?

What was it you most enjoyed?

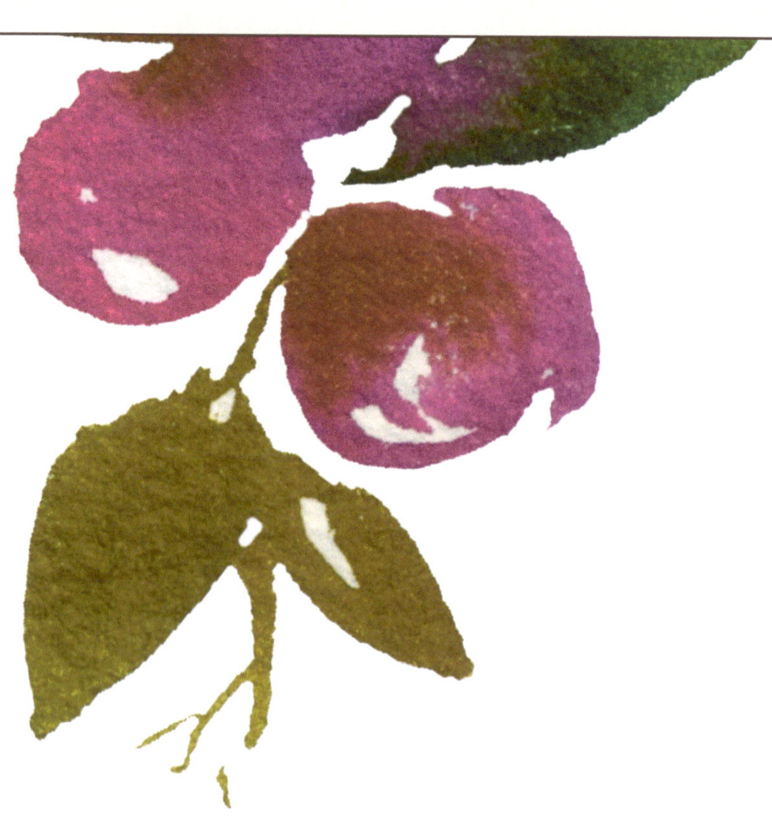

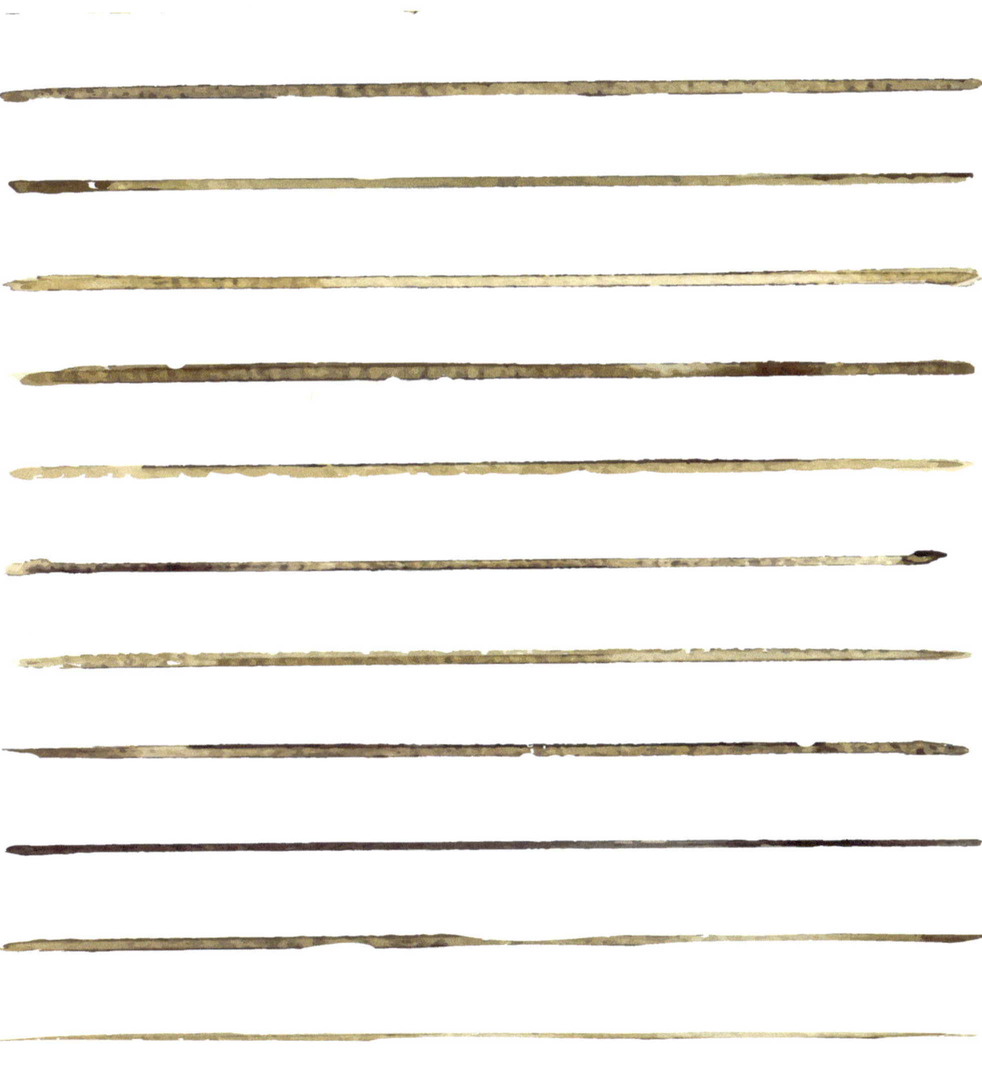
Day 28

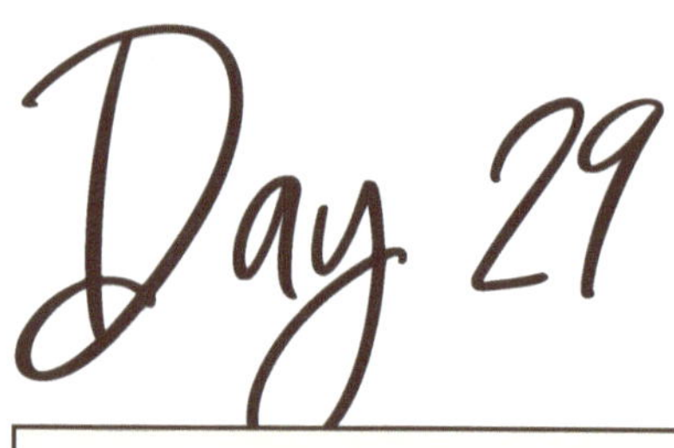

What family tradition do you love?

Who in your family started it?

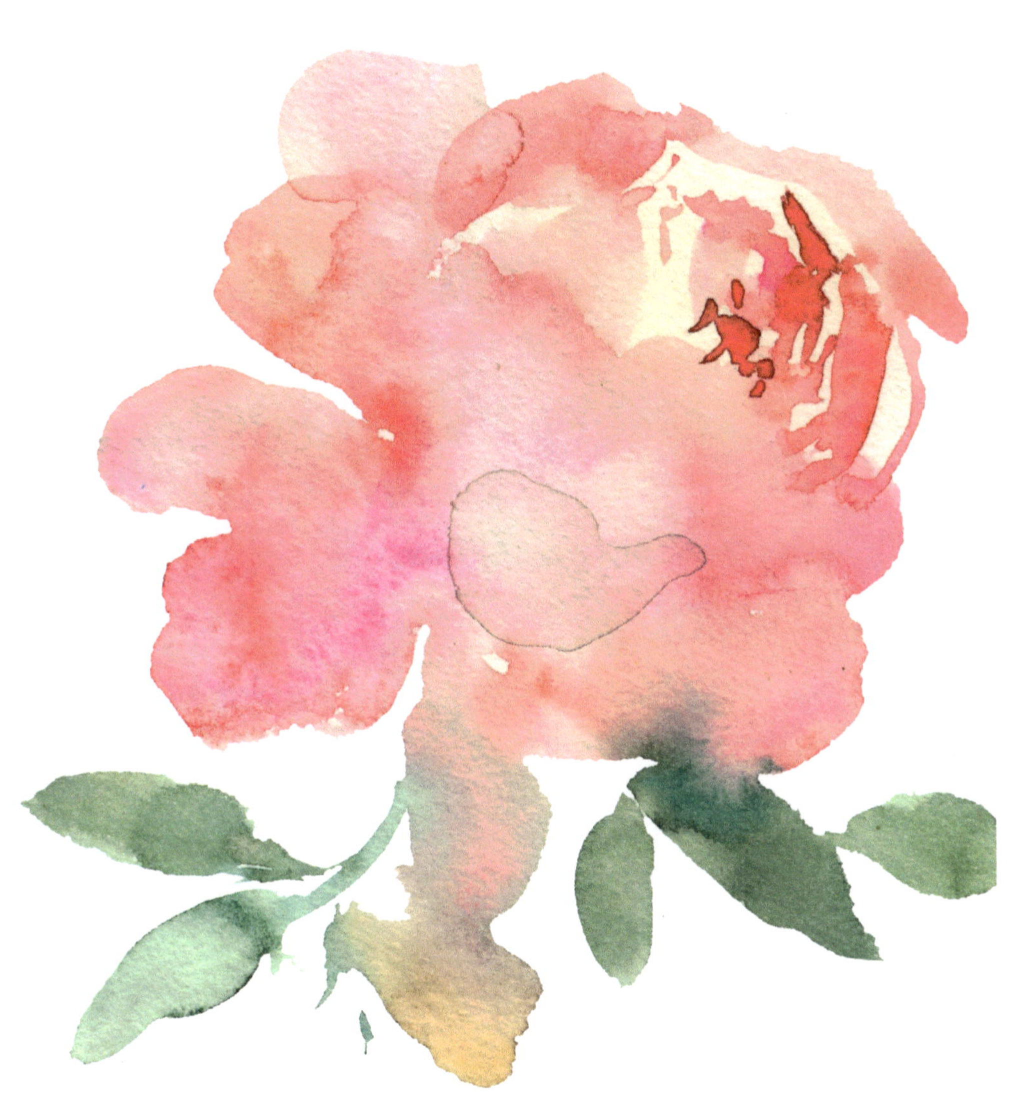

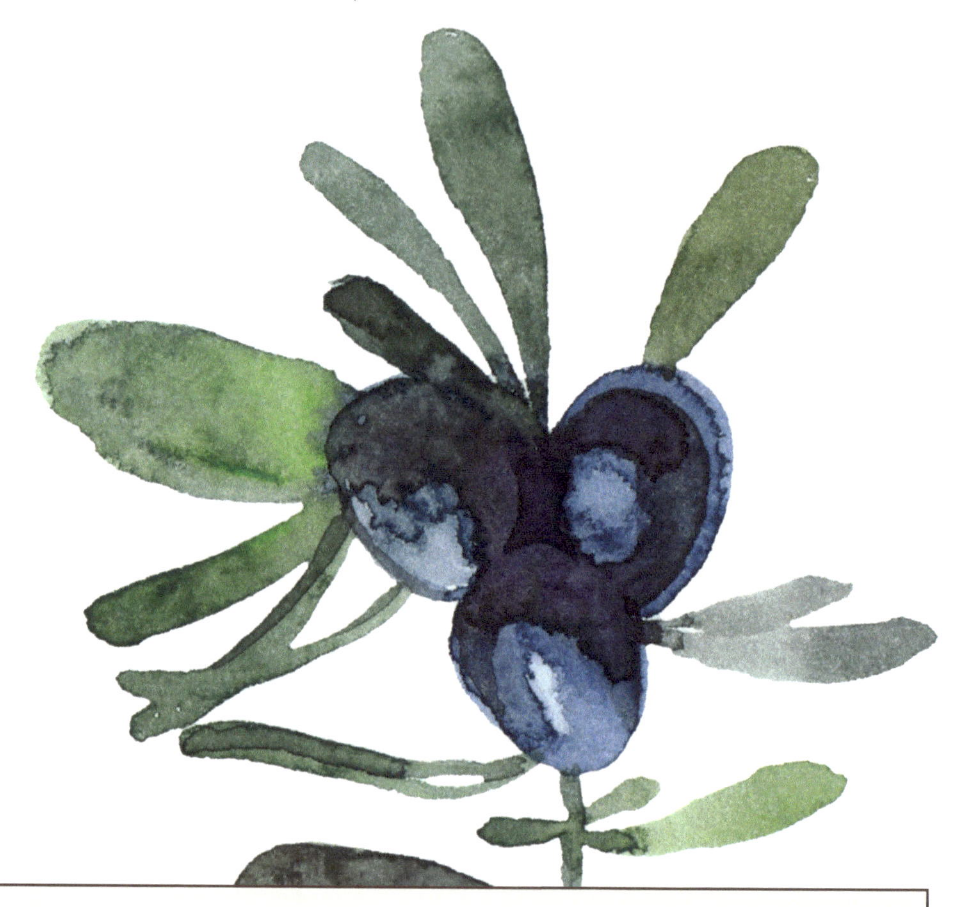

What is your favorite Dad joke?

Whose dad told it?

Day 30

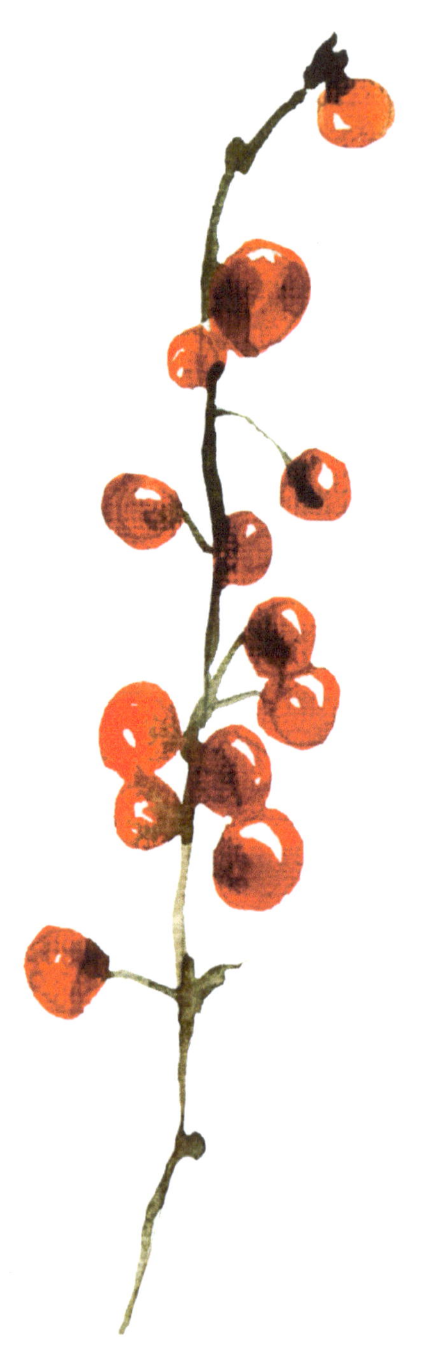

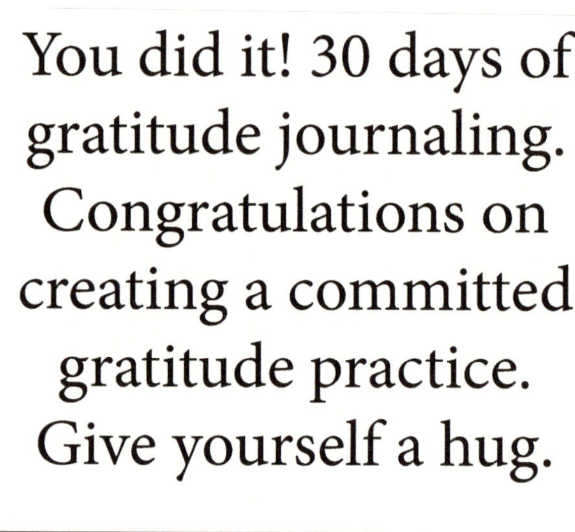

You did it! 30 days of gratitude journaling. Congratulations on creating a committed gratitude practice. Give yourself a hug.

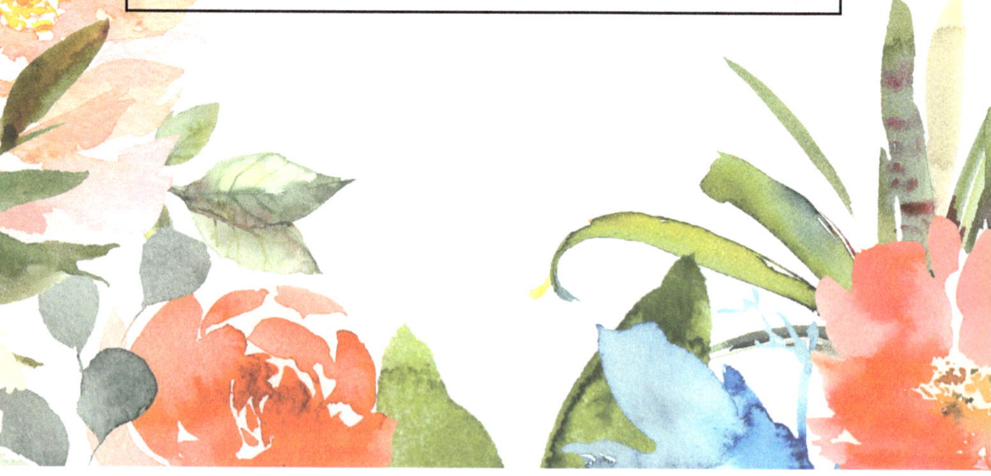

If you enjoyed this book please consider leaving a review on the details page.
Contact me at tk@trinakay.com with questions or suggestions for a new book. Thank you for taking this journey with me. - Grace and peace, Trina Kay